Ernst Schering Research Foundation Workshop
Supplement 8
New Pharmacological Approaches to Reproductive Health and Healthy Ageing

Springer
Berlin
Heidelberg
New York
Barcelona
Hong Kong
London
Milan
Paris
Tokyo

Ernst Schering Research Foundation Workshop
Supplement 8

New Pharmacological Approaches to Reproductive Health and Healthy Ageing

Symposium on the Occasion of the 80th Birthday of Professor Egon Diczfalusy

Werner-Karl Raff, Mahmoud F. Fathalla,
Farid Saad
Editors

With 19 Figures and 9 Tables

Springer

Series Editors: G. Stock and M. Lessl

ISSN 1431-7133
ISBN 3-540-42234-X Springer-Verlag Berlin Heidelberg New York

Die Deutsche Bibliothek – CIP-Einheitsaufnahme
New pharmacological approaches to reproductive health and healthy ageing : with tables / Symposium on the occasion of the 80th birthday of Professor Egon Diczfalusy. Ernst Schering Research Foundation. Ed.: Werner-Karl Raff ... - Berlin ; Heidelberg ; New York ; Barcelona ; Hongkong ; London ; Milan ; Paris ; Singapore ; Tokyo : Springer, 2001
(Ernst Schering Research Foundation Workshop : Supplement ; 8)
ISBN 3-540-42234-X

Springer-Verlag Berlin Heidelberg New York
a member of BertelsmannSpringer Science+Business Media GmbH

http://www.springer.de

Printed in Germany

Typesetting: Data conversion by Springer-Verlag
Printing: Druckhaus Beltz, Hemsbach.
Binding: J. Schäffer GmbH & Co. KG, Grünstadt
SPIN:10842535 21/3130/AG–5 4 3 2 1 0 – Printed on acid-free paper

Preface

In honour of the 80th birthday of Egon Diczfalusy, the Ernst Schering Research Foundation organized a scientific workshop entitled "Farewell to the 20th Century: New Pharmacological Approaches to Reproductive Health and Healthy Ageing" in Berlin on 1–2 October 2000.

Egon Diczfalusy was born in Miskolc, Hungary, on 19 September 1920. Eighty years later, it was Egon Diczfalusy, MD, PhD, DSc(hon.), Dr.h.c.(mult.), FRCOG, FACOG (hon.), Professor emeritus, Karolinska Institutet, Stockholm, who took active part in the workshop. He was accompanied by his wife Ann, their daughter and four sons. The workshop elicited a great interest worldwide; its programme might be understood as a turn-of-the century reflection of the lifework of Diczfalusy, the great communicator. Hence, the workshop covered a very broad area of subjects from the current state of analytics via biochemistry and physiology, as well as clinical use of sex hormones via family planning and hormone replacement therapy for the human male and female, to a discussion of the new challenge of the new century: a gradual increase in the proportion of elderly people combined with a gradual decrease in the proportion of younger people both in developed and developing countries.

The manifold scientific presentations and the sometimes (fortunately) controversial round table discussions were both informative and stimulating. The overwhelming majority of the many outstanding speakers were recruited from Egon's friends and former disciples from all corners of the world. One of them, Prof. Benagiano outlining Egon Diczfalusy's life, described him as one of the last exponents of the past century's remarkable generalists and grand seigneurs. Egon was born

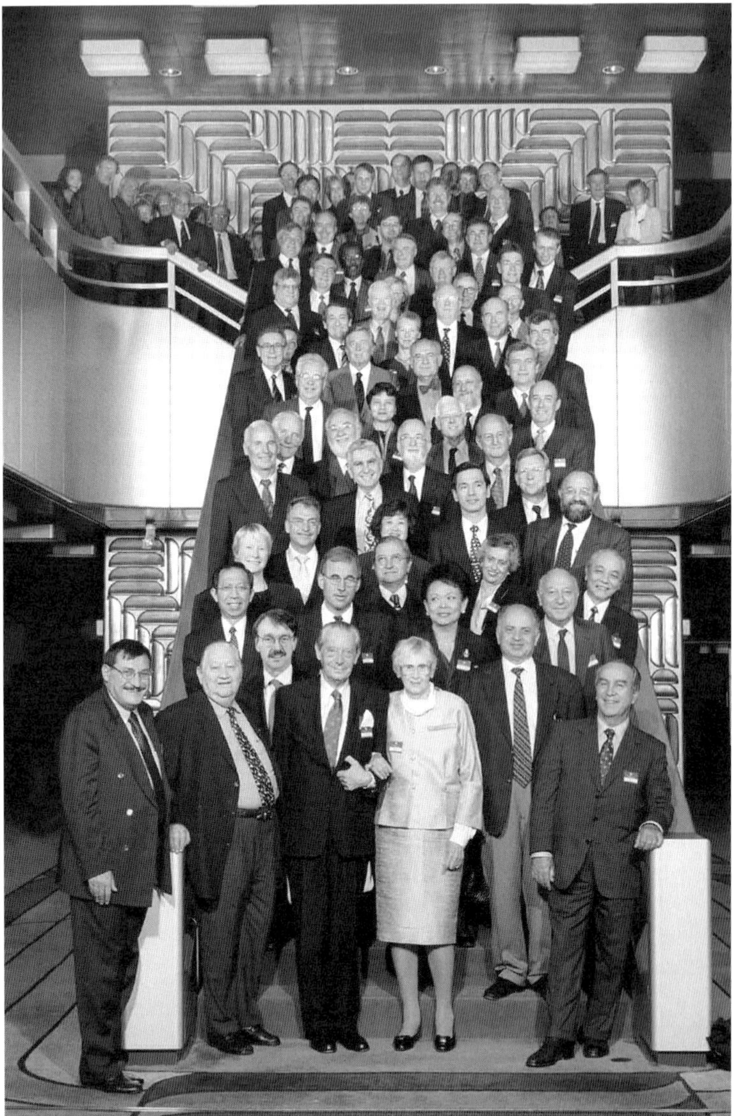

The participants of the workshop

with the – in him it is still prevailing – spirit of the old multicultural and multiethnic Austro-Hungarian monarchy. Later, the generously equipped and cosmopolitan Karolinska Institute in Stockholm became the environment of his scientific maturation. Diczfalusy was one of the principal initiators of the Human Reproduction Programme of the World Health Organization some 30 years ago; he was always deeply committed to progress in reproductive endocrinology and was (and still is) profoundly convinced of the necessity of an active and long-lasting scientific support of the Third World. Even today, he is very active as a scientific mentor and reliable friend of a large number of reproductive endocrinologists and clinicians all over the world. He has an unerring eye for what is required in developing countries. He is politically alert and has outstanding organizational skills.

It is a particular honour and privilege for us to publish the proceedings of the workshop in the prestigious series of publications of the Ernst Schering Research Foundation.

Werner-Karl Raff, Mahmoud F. Fathalla, Farid Saad

Contents

List of Editors and Contributors

Editors

Raff, W.K.
Strategic Business Unit, Fertility Control and Hormone Therapy, Schering AG, Müllerstrasse 178, 13342 Berlin, Germany

Fathalla, M.F.
The Rockefeller Foundation, Biomedical and Reproductive Health Research and Training, P.O. Box 30, Assiut, Egypt

Saad, F.
Strategic Business Unit, Fertility Control and Hormone Therapy, Schering AG, Müllerstrasse 178, 13342 Berlin, Germany

Contributors

Affandi, B.
Klinik Raden Saleh Raya, Subdivision of Reproductive Health, Department of Obstetrics and Gynaecology, University of Jakarta, Jalan Raden Saleh Raya 49, Jakarta 10330, Indonesia

Archer, D.F.
CONRAD Clinical Research Center, The Jones Institute for Reproduction, 601 Colley Avenue, Norfolk, VA 23505, USA

Aso, T.
Department of Obstetrics and Gynecology, Tokyo Medical and Dental University, Faculty of Medicine, 1-5-45 Yushima, Bunkyo-ku, Tokyo 113-8519, Japan

Baird, D.T.
Centre for Reproductive Biology, Department of Obstetrics and Gynaecology, 37 Chalmers Street, Edinburgh EH3 9EW, UK

Balogh, À.
Department of Obstetrics and Gynecology, University of Debrecen, Medical and Health Sciences Center, P.O. Box 37, 4012 Debrecen, Hungary

Benagiano, G.
Istituto Superiore di Sanità, Viale Regina Elena, 299, 00161 Rome, Italy

Bialy, G.
Center for Population Research, National Institute of Health, Executive Building, Suite 8 B 07, 6100 Executive Boulevard, Bethesda, MD 20892-7510, USA

Brinkmann, A.O.
Department of Endocrinology and Reproduction, Erasmus University Rotterdam, P.O. Box 1738, 3000 DR Rotterdam, The Netherlands

Boonkasemsanti, W.
Department of Obstetrics and Gynaecology, Faculty of Medicine, Chulalongkorn University, Rama IV Road, Bangkok 10330, Thailand

Cato, A.C.B.
Forschungszentrum Karlsruhe, Institute of Toxicology and Genetics, Weberstrasse 5, 76133 Karlsruhe, Germany

Crosignani, P.G.
Clinica Ostetrica E Ginecologica I, Facoltà Di Medicina E Chirurgia, Via Commenda, 12, 20429 Milano, Italy

Croxatto, H.B.
Instituto Chileno de Medicina Reproductiva, Jose Ramon Gutierrez 295 Depto. 3, Casilla 96 Correo 22, Santiago, Chile

Diczfalusy, E.
Rönningevägen 21, 14461Rönninge, Sweden

Gabelnick, H.L.
CONRAD Program, 1611 North Kent Street, Suite 806, Arlington, VA 22209, USA

Herbert, J.
Department of Anatomy, University of Cambridge, Downing Street, Cambridge CB2 3DY, UK

Hoshiai, H.
Department of Obstetrics and Gynaecology, Kinki University School of Medicine, 377-2 Ohno-Higashi, Osaka-Sayama, Osaka 589-0014, Japan

Ivell, R.
Institute for Hormone and Fertility Research, Grandweg 64, 22529 Hamburg, Germany

Jänne, O.A.
Professor of Physiology, Director, Biomedicum Helsinki, University of Helsinki, P.O. Box 9 (Siltavuorenpenger 20 J), 00014 Helsinki, Finland

Kalache, A.
Ageing and Health Programme, World Health Organization, 20 Avenue Appia, 1211 Geneva 27, Switzerland

Keller, I.
Ageing and Health Programme, World Health Organization, 20 Avenue Appia, 1211 Geneva 27, Switzerland

Kovács, L.
Department of Obstetrics and Gynaecology, Albert Szent-Györgyi Medical University, Semmelweis u. 1, 6725 Szeged, Hungary

Limpaphayom, K.K.
Department of Obstetrics and Gynaecology, Faculty of Medicine, Chulalongkorn University, Rama IV Road, Pathumwan, Bangkok 10330, Thailand

Mancuso, S.
Direttore, Istituto di Clinica Ostetrica e Ginecologica, Università Cattolica del Sacro Cuore, Policlinico Gemelli, Largo A. Gemelli, 1, 00168 Rome, Italy

Martini, L.
Department of Endocrinology, University of Milan, Via Balzaretti 9, 20133 Milan, Italy

Mittelstrass, J.
Philosophische Fakultät, Universität Konstanz, Universitätsstrasse 10, 78457 Konstanz, Germany

Naftolin, F.
Yale University School of Medicine, Department of Obstetrics and Gynecology, 333 Cedar Street, 335 FMB, New Haven, CT 06520, USA

Oelkers, W.
Freie Universität Berlin, Klinikum Benjamin Franklin, Abteilung Endokrinologie, Hindenburgdamm 30, 12200 Berlin, Germany

Rivier, C.
Clayton Foundation, Laboratory of Peptide Biology, Salk Institute, 10010 North Torrey Pines Road, San Diego, CA 92037, USA

Schneider, H.P.G.
Universitäts-Frauenklinik, Albert-Schweitzer-Strasse 33, 48148 Münster, Germany

Segars, J.H.
Developmental Endocrinology Branch, National Institute of Child Health and Human Development, Bethesda, MD 20892, USA

Stock, G.
Schering Research Foundation, Müllerstrasse 178, 13342 Berlin, Germany

Swerdloff, R.S.
Division of Endocrinology, Department of Med/Endo, Bldg. RB1, Harbor-UCLA Medical Center/Room 229, 1124 West Carson Street, Torrance, CA 90502-2006, USA

Telegdy, G.
University of Szeged, Faculty of General Medicine, Albert Szent-Györgyi Medical and Pharmaceutical Center, Department of Pathophysiology, Semmelweis St. 1, 6725 Szeged, Hungary

1 Laudation
Presenting Professor Egon Diczfalusy on his 80th Birthday

G. Benagiano

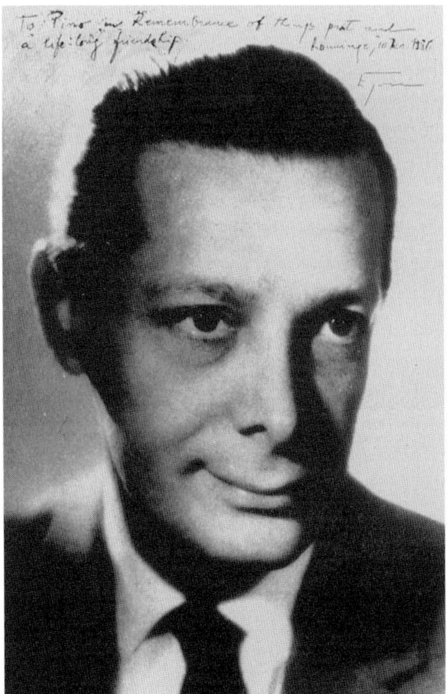

Fig. 1. Prof. Egon Diczfalusy circa 1967

To retrace the life and many accomplishments of Egon Diczfalusy (Fig. 1) on the occasion of his 80th birthday is at the same time a very simple and an almost impossible task. It is simple because I have been associated with him for more than 37 years and because I am talking to his closest friends and associates: most of you have known him for years, have shared good and perhaps even bad moments with him and are well acquainted with the milestones in his life. It is a very complex, almost impossible endeavour because his personality has so many facets that it is very hard to do him justice outlining all of them, even when you have known him for so long.

For this reason, on the one hand I cannot avoid sketching the composite picture of the man and scientist, of the person dedicated to the progress of humanity and to its liberation from all kinds of evils; on the other, I must try to give you a sort of "inside" look into the more personal aspects of his life. In order to do so, I am afraid that, in presenting him, instead of a stuffy laudation, I will provide you with a slightly irreverent, although most affectionate description of a man who played such a unique role in my life, second only to my own father.

Egon Diczfalusy's life can probably be said to encompass four major epochs: the first starts in his native Hungary and ends in 1946 when he, later followed by his mother, moved to Sweden. The second, comprises his heroic days in Sweden – the most productive part of his life – when the foeto-placental unit was discovered and carefully researched. The third spans some 25 years and begins when he, together with Alex Kessler and with the help of the Ford Foundation, conceived the WHO Expanded Programme of Research in Human Reproduction, which later developed into the Special Programme of Research, Development and Research Training in Human Reproduction (the mythical HRP), co-sponsored by UNDP, UNFPA, WHO and the World Bank; and the fourth reaches to our days when, as he himself aged, he turned his attention to an ageing humanity, quickly becoming – typical of the way he proceeds – a real expert.

Of his "first life", which I will name the Hungarian time, we know little; however, some of the stories we heard in Stockholm some 35 years ago provide intriguing flashes into the life of the Hungarian military establishment to which his family belonged, thanks to his father, a General (Fig. 2). It was the time between the two World Wars, a special period for Hungary, that of independence from Austria.

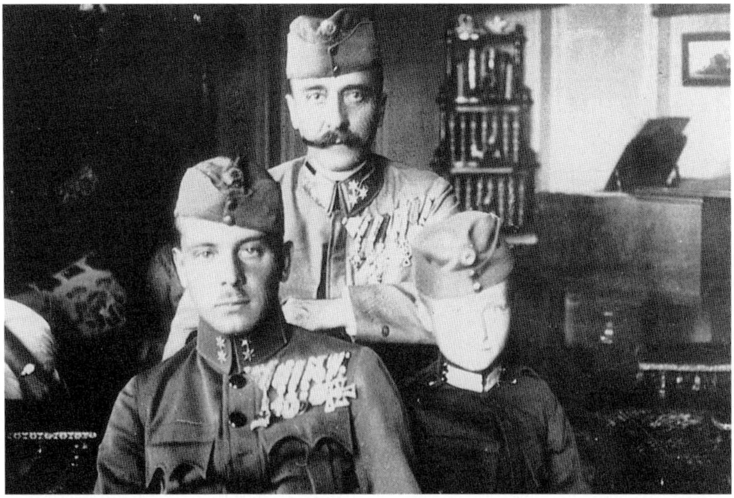

Fig. 2. Diczfalusy's grandfather (*back*) at age 54 (1918 in Košice, Slovakia); Diczfalusy's father (*front left*) aged 23; Diczfalusy's uncle (*front right*), aged 11

Allow me to share two little anecdotes, which he told us many years ago and which I hope he still remembers: the first is the story of an officer who took the Orient Express all the way to Istanbul to buy flowers for the lady he had just met and fallen in love with; the second is the story of the officer who became a regular guest at lunch, each day for a month, in his paternal house, the reason being that he had spent all his salary to celebrate in a café – inviting all those who happened to be present – his beautiful new love!

It was this cultural milieu which helped forge his personality in his native Miskolc, a small city in north-eastern Hungary (Fig. 3a), and subsequently during his medical school days at the Semmelweis University in Szeged (Fig. 3b), in the very south of Hungary, where he graduated summa cum laude. An Italian proverb recites, "If you start well, you are already mid-way."

Less than 2 years later, he moved to Sweden where the second phase of his life started, the one I will call the Swedish time. His first teacher in his new homeland, back in 1946, was a Nobel laureate, Prof. Hans

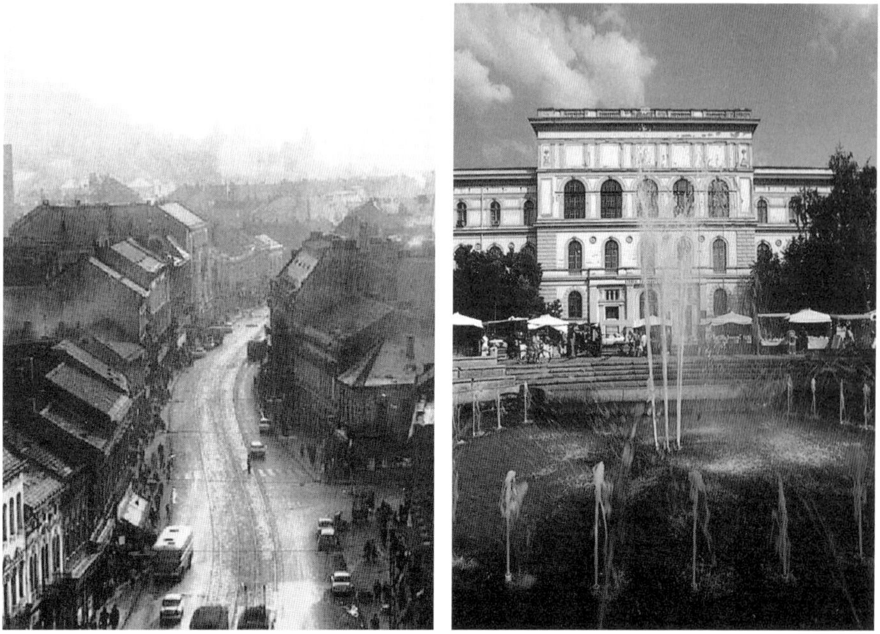

A **Fig. 3. A** Miskolc, Diczfalusy's birthplace. **B** Main building, Semmelweis University in Szeged, where Diczfalusy graduated summa cum laude B

Von Euler (see Fig. 4a), whom Egon knew for a very specific reason, as I will tell you in a minute.

He soon moved to Kvinnokliniken, The Department of Women's Diseases, under the direction of Prof. Axel Westman (see Fig. 4b), where in 1953, he completed his thesis on "Chorionic Gonadotropin and Oestrogens in the Human Placenta" (Diczfalusy 1953), to become Dozent (the equivalent of a PhD) and, at the same time, Associate Professor of Experimental Endocrinology. From then on, the main focus of his scientific work became the hormones involved in human reproduction.

When I met Egon Diczfalusy in 1963, he had just been awarded one of the largest Ford Foundation Grants in Reproductive Endocrinology of those days: half a million dollars to study steroid biogenesis and metabolism in the human foetus, placenta and maternal organism.

A 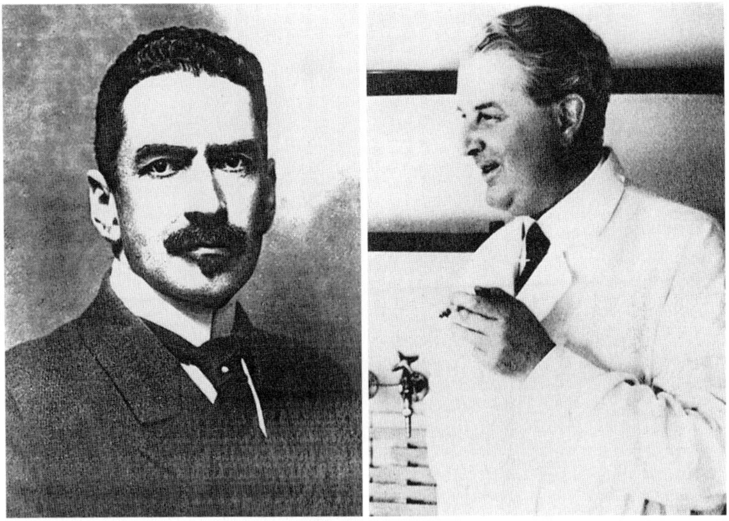 B

Fig. 4. A Nobel laureate Prof. Hans Von Euler was Diczfalusy's first teacher in Sweden. **B** Prof. Axel Westman

Through hard work and fighting difficult conditions (a foreigner has always difficulties in adjusting to a new country), he had become the Laborator, or Head, of the Hormonlaboratoriet at the Karolinska Sjukhuset, or Karolinska Hospital.

When, in 1978, Egon recalled the early days of reproductive endocrinology in giving the Sir Henry Dale Lecture, he called this period "the merry post-war days". There is one section in this lecture that I must recall for you because it contains a lot of insight into his early life. Egon wrote: "How did I become a reproductive endocrinologist? By the Hungarian approach. As a second year medical student at the University of Szeged, Hungary, I was working in the Department of Pathology and Bacteriology of Prof. Györgyi Ivánovics and my first task was to repeat a study by the Nobel laureate, Hans von Euler and his co-workers in Stockholm, who found transaminase activity in suspensions of yeast and *E. coli* bacilli. I just could not confirm their findings, and my professor felt that I must publish this. This negative report was my first publication; it was probably instrumental in bringing me to Stockholm after the

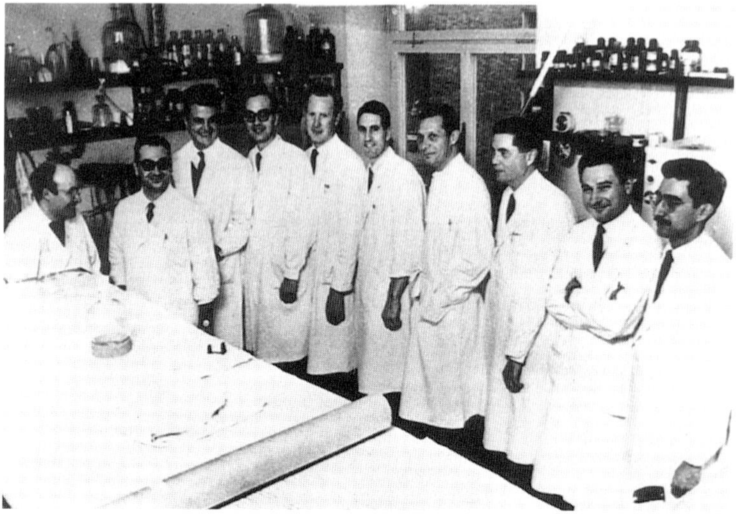

Fig. 5. One of the early groups of visiting scientists present at the Hormonlaboratoriet immediately after the Ford Foundation awarded its grant

war, when I had the privilege to work as Prof. Hans von Euler's assistant during the years 1946–1947" (Diczfalusy 1978).

As you can see everything fits!

The old Hormonlaboratoriet, as well as the new one, has become famous for the number of young (and not so young) visiting scientists who trained there from all over the world (Fig. 5): Diczfalusy's own curriculum states that some 150 scientists trained at Karolinska under him, a good half coming from developing countries. A couple of dozen, including two of his Italian graduate students, eventually became chairmen of university departments scattered in the four corners of the world.

Those were hectic days of hard work, but also great satisfaction. I remember the first time we all went to an international meeting in Hamburg, an Acta Endocrinologica Congress. One of my friends from Italy ventured to be the first of the group to give his paper (Dell'Acqua et al. 1965); at the end he went to see Egon to receive his comments, and all Egon said was: "Sergio, you had better improve your English, if you want to ever present a paper again." No kidding! With this preamble, I still remember that I did not sleep that night; I swore to myself I would learn English and learn it well and, to achieve this, I even married an English-speaking lady!

I want to take this opportunity to reveal a little secret kept for 35 years. You may laugh at it, but at the time this little joke was considered "desecration". The inside of the laboratory's toilet bore a small sign that read: "Efter toalet besöket, alltid twätta händerna", that is, "After visiting the toilet always remember to wash your hands". But one terrible day the "h" in the word "händerna", or "the hands", had been covered with medical white tape and the word now read "änderna", that is, "your ass". In reality it was plural (your asses) – bad Swedish, perhaps, but nevertheless perfectly understandable! Egon was furious and wanted to know who had dared to be so impertinent. Well Egon, I am afraid it was your demure, studious-looking, young Italian pupil, Pino Benagiano. I hope you are now ready to pardon me.

As I have mentioned, Diczfalusy's scientific production started in 1942 when he was a second year medical student (Diczfalusy 1942); his first paper dealing with steroids appeared in 1948 (Aldman et al. 1948). Today his production amounts to more than 620 publications; he is the editor of some 30 books and has been the series editor of both the *Karolinska Symposia on Research Methods in Reproductive Endocrinology*, published between 1969 and 1975 and distributed to 10,000 people, and *Vitamins and Hormones* between 1970 and 1982. This prolific time, the years of the definition of the foeto-placental unit, was certainly his most productive, and Diczfalusy's papers became landmarks in *Acta Endocrinologica*. To represent this epoch, I wish to remember one paper, "Oestriol Metabolism at Midpregnancy" (Diczfalusy and Benagiano 1966), for two reasons: first, because my name appears next to his, and second, because it deals with the metabolism of the one steroid that really requires the foeto-placental unit to be synthesized: oestriol.

Notwithstanding the vast number of papers produced in those days, he personally typed each first draft on a little typewriter in his office, re-writing each sentence until he was satisfied that all the data had been put on paper.

In spite of being exigent, he really cared for all of us; he was sort of jealous of letting each of us go our own way. When – after receiving a good offer from the Population Council in New York – I decided to leave, he summoned me to his office and asked bluntly: "Are you going

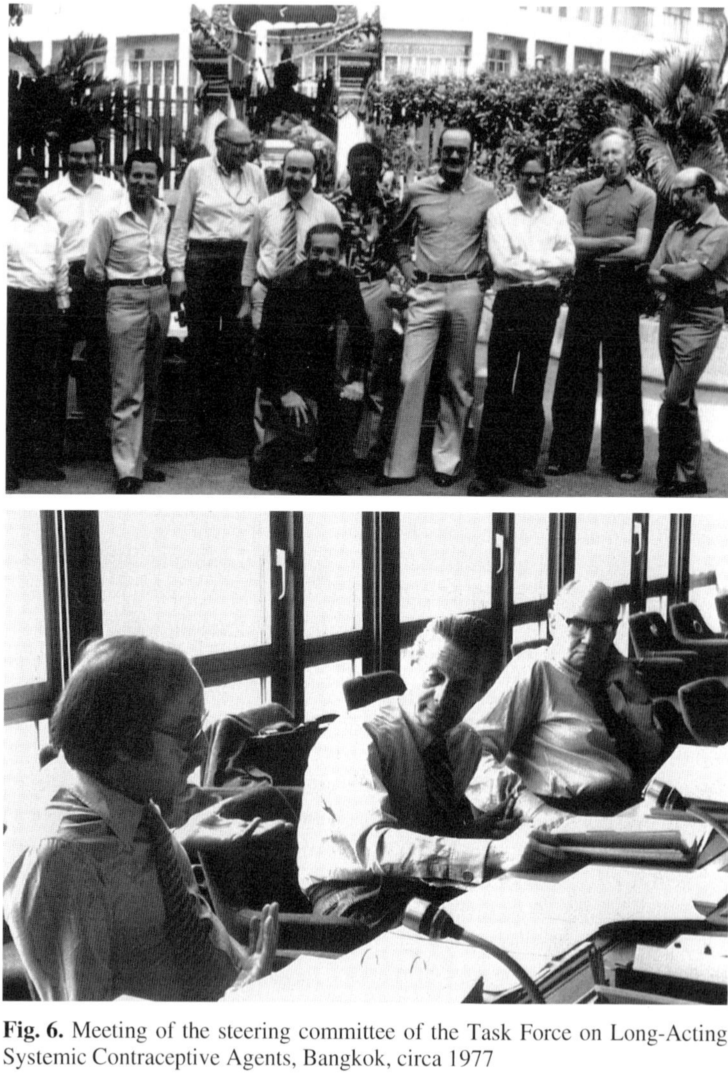

Fig. 6. Meeting of the steering committee of the Task Force on Long-Acting Systemic Contraceptive Agents, Bangkok, circa 1977

because you will get a better salary, or because you like the type of research better, or because you will be able to do better politicking?" And I smiled innocently and said: "But of course all three sir!" I left because I had to leave, but I left my heart there (if you want the whole truth, both in terms of scientific interest and in terms of sentimental attachment). For these two reasons I kept in close contact with him, the laboratory and Sverige. So did many others, and the Swedish Mafia that he created there is – to this day – a solid group of friend scientists who learned at a severe and demanding school and who spread this new creed all over the world.

The "third life" of Egon Diczfalusy, which I will call the Swiss connection, brought him the world dimension and perspective for which he is famous today: I am sure the seven languages he can speak easily helped him in dealing with WHO; however, it is his personality, his knowledge and his dedication that made him indispensable to four consecutive Human Reproduction Programme Directors there, as Senior Consultant. Since then he has been on every major task force steering committee (Fig. 6), while at the same time heading the WHO Collaborating Centre in Research and Research Training in Stockholm, travelling on behalf of the Organization more than any other person I know and participating in more conferences and workshops than probably any one in this audience.

During 25 years, his advice to the Programme has been invaluable and his knowledge of the work carried out by it unsurpassed. For this reason when José Barzelatto decided that the Programme's first 15 years should be celebrated with a document summarizing the many accomplishments made, he turned to Egon Diczfalusy, who took the task with enthusiasm and thoroughness. I will only quote one sentence which summarizes his view on the role of international co-operation: "A modern interpretation of history is said to be based on the analysis of the history of ideas. The history of the second part of the twentieth century represents an entirely new departure in this respect; for the first time in the history of mankind, the policies emerging from world conferences organized by the various specialized agencies of the United Nations broadened the views and perceptions of many member states (including donor governments) and significantly influenced their policies" (Diczfalusy 1986).

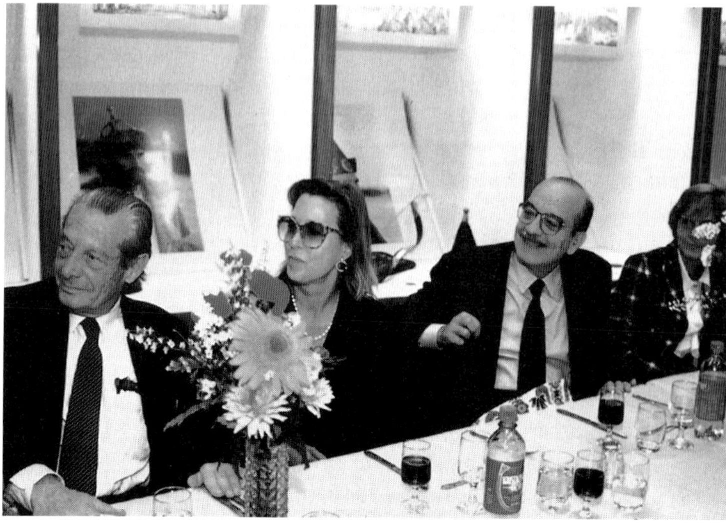

Fig. 7. The celebration of the 25th anniversary of HRP. *From left to right*, E. Diczfalusy, Mrs. Benagiano, G. Benagiano and Mrs. Ann Diczfalusy

It is also thanks to his indefatigable efforts that we were able to celebrate the Programme's 25th birthday in 1997 in Szeged, his home city (Kovács and Resch 1998). Summarizing these first 25 years was, in fact, my last duty as Director of the Special Programme, although, I had actually formally resigned 3 months earlier to return to Rome. In opening the celebrations, Egon challenged all of us by saying: "I myself represent the future. Yes, you heard right, I said the future. I represent the future of the past. As Paul Valéry puts it: 'Are you not the future of all memories stored within you? The future of the past'" (Diczfalusy 1998). And I want this to be the motto of this Symposium: we are here to celebrate above all the future of the past.

The celebration of the 25th anniversary of HRP was uniquely important to me, not only as my swan song as HRP director, but also because László Kóvacs and his collaborators concocted a special celebration for my 60th birthday (Fig. 7). I can only dream of what the celebration for my 80th birthday will be with Egon giving the laudation, although, with my five bypasses, I should – as Egon often says – minimize my expectations. We shall see!

His work with WHO brought him more and more often to Geneva, where he sort of took up residence in my apartment. Those were pleasant and busy days and we travelled together many times, often fighting over being late for planes: I remember once when we went to Palo Alto, renting a car at San Francisco Airport. About two-and-a-half hours before the plane's departure he became uneasy and wanted to leave. I reassured him that by taking the Junipero Sierra Freeway and speeding up a little bit we could finish our business and still be at the airport half-an-hour before departure, but he was not satisfied. At the end I gave up and we left, arriving at the airport fairly early (at least by my standards); so I told him: "Do you see? We are here 40 minutes before departure"; he looked at me scornfully and said: "Don't you know that the gate opens 50 minutes before departure?" In this sense, Egon should have married my wife and together they could happily go and...as I say, open up the airport in the morning.

As a little song of the Wolf Cubs goes: "Everything ends in this world" and even the HRP days ended for Egon. When he turned 75, Dario Sanvincenti, the Director of Personnel, informed me that he was forced to stop the consultancy agreement with Egon Diczfalusy. This, however, would not preclude his working as an advisor, and – of course – that's exactly what he did. With one caveat: he started advising the WHO Programme on Ageing, as well as the Rockefeller Foundation.

In a way, I am glad Sanvincenti did what he did, because it helped this "young 75-year-old" start a new career and the fourth and present phase in his life, which I will call the world time, not because he wasn't in the world arena before; rather, because he now is truly the epitome of a world citizen.

As a matter of fact, I was among the first to benefit from this new phase of his life: FIGO, the International Federation of Gynecology and Obstetrics, had asked me to write a chapter for the Second World Report on Women's Health and gave me women's longevity as the theme (Diczfalusy and Benagiano 1997). I was buried in work and had no way to amass all the evidence, all the data necessary to write something meaningful. So I turned to Egon, who basically sent me a ready-to-print manuscript to which I had little to add, except my name, of course.

I will only quote a couple of sentences from his latest papers because they are recent and because his thinking in this field is still evolving. I will tell you more about it when we meet in 10 years' time!

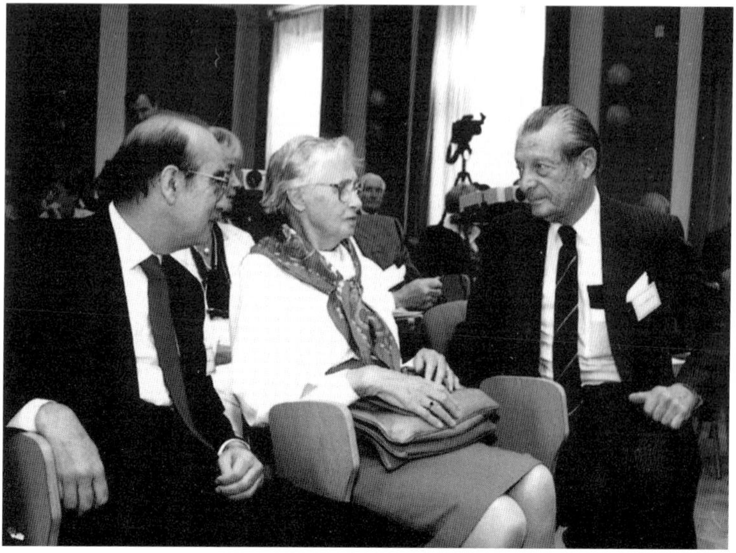

Fig. 8. Mrs. Ann Diczfalusy between E. Diczfalusy (*right*) and Benagiano, in Szeged, 1997

Recently, in a main article in the *International Journal of Gynecology and Obstetrics* he wrote: "The wind of new realities is blowing with increasing strength. It is up to us to decide whether we prefer protective windscreens or new types of windmills" (Diczfalusy E 1999a). Clearly, Egon has never cherished protective windscreens; he has always been out where "the action is".

His life has been dedicated to achieve what – and, again I quote from one of his latest papers – Arnold Toynbee remarked: "Our time is the first since the dawn of civilization in which people have dared to think it practicable to make the benefits of civilization available to the whole human race" (Diczfalusy 1999b). Indeed, as a faithful pupil, I have been saying that the true challenge for public health in the twenty-first century is not to apply the knowledge arising from sequencing the human genome or from other frontier discoveries; rather it is to provide to the entire human race the kind of health care already available today to a privileged small minority.

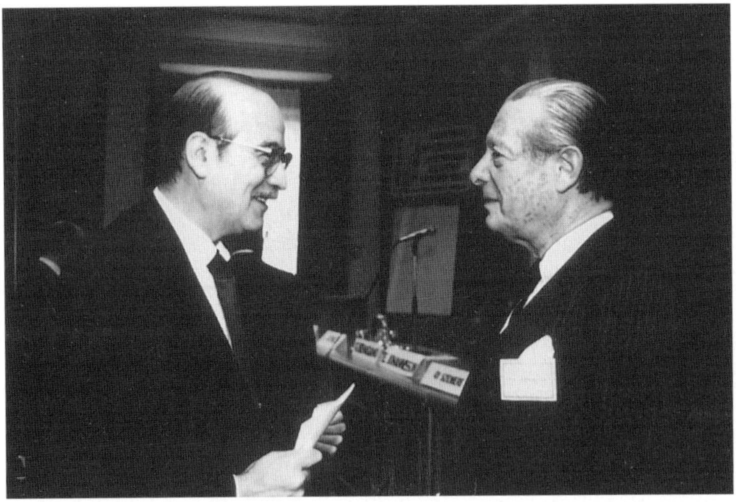

Fig. 9. Diczfalusy (*right*) receiving congratulations from Benagiano

The real challenge is – to use the Latin sentence with which he closed another leading article published this year – to do so "*in nomine dignitatis, scientiae et charitatis*" (Diczfalusy 2000), in the name of human dignity, science and love.

Well, I was given only 30 minutes and, therefore, must finish this laudation. I can only do so apologizing for not having been able to do Egon justice, to provide you with a full picture of the man we are honouring here today; but that would have – of course – been simply impossible. I do hope, though, to have given you an idea not only of his achievements, of his dedication to the world of science, as well as to human suffering; not only an idea of how much he cared for his pupils, as well as for every couple on the earth needing help to cope with their family problems; but also an idea of the man behind the scientist, of the master and the friend of a lifetime. And allow me to paraphrase what the American magazine *Life* said about the Romans in a famous series published over 20 years ago (Life 8.8, 1966) and say: I tried to give you an idea of the man who shaped and forever changed my life.

There is, however, one very last (but certainly not least) mention I must make; in Italy we say, Behind every great man there is a great woman. Nothing could be more true: Ann's influence on Egon has been enormous; more often than not, trying to calm him down, and God only knows if he needed it! She was the point of reference to always go back to; caring for children and grand children; withstanding drama and even tragedy, but always there, whenever she was needed. Thanks, Ann, for taking on the impossible job: to be his wife!

And it is with affection and pride that I conclude by way of a simple statement by Leonardo da Vinci: "*Tristo è quel discepolo che non supera il suo maestro*", that is: Wicked is the disciple who does not excel over his master. Well, Egon, old fellah, this statement has always been a thorn in my flesh. Here I have miserably failed; as a matter of fact, we all failed, since no one among us has been able to excel over you.

On my part I, I wish you the classic "one hundred of these birthdays" (Fig. 9) and at the same time I can only swear that I will continue to try, but with little hope, to at least come close to my friend and mentor, Egon Diczfalusy, Prof. Emeritus at Karolinska Institute in Stockholm.

References

Diczfalusy E (1953) Chorionic gonadotrophin and oestrogens on the human placenta. Acta Endocr (Kbh) Suppl 12

Diczfalusy E (1978) Reproductive endocrinology and the merry post-war years. J Endocrinol 79:1–17

Dell'Acqua S, Mancuso S, Eriksson G, Diczfalusy E (1965) Estrogen formation from 19-nor-testosterone and testosterone following in situ perfusion of human placental at midterm. 5th Acta Endocrinological Congress Abstract n.49. Acta Endocrinol (Copenh) Suppl 100:81

Diczfalusy E (1942) Die Frage der Umaminierung durch Bacterienzellen. Biochem Z 313:75–76

Aldman B, Diczfalusy E, Rosenberg T (1948) In vitro inhibition of alkaline phosphatase by estrogenic hormones. Acta Chem Scand 2:529–530

Diczfalusy E, Benagiano G (1966) Oestriol metabolism at mid-pregnancy. Res Steroids 2:27–45

Diczfalusy E (1986) World Health Organization. Special programme of research, development and research training in human reproduction. The first fifteen years: a review. Contraception 34:3–119

Kovács L, Resch BA (1998) Research on Human Reproduction. Albert Szent-Györgyi Medical University Press, Szeged

Diczfalusy E (1998) The contraceptive revolution: its past and future "history". In: Kovács L, Resch BA (eds) Research on Human Reproduction. Albert Szent-Györgyi Medical University Press, Szeged, pp 23–35

Diczfalusy E, Benagiano G (1997) Women and the third and fourth age. Int J Obstet Gynecol 58:177–188

Diczfalusy E (1999a) The past, present and future. Int J Gynecol Obstet 67(Suppl 2):153–157

Diczfalusy E (1999b) From the contraceptive to the anthropocentric revolution (Gregory Pincus, in Memoriam). Eur J Contracept Reprod Health Care 4:187–201

Diczfalusy E (2000) The contraceptive revolution. Contraception 6(1):3–7

2 Ageing in the Twenty-first Century

A. Kalache, I. Keller

1 Introduction

One of the main features of the world population within the next few decades will be the rapid increase in the absolute and relative numbers of older people in both developing and developed countries. We are right now at the threshold of global ageing. The total number of elderly people (defined as 60 years of age and older) worldwide is expected to increase from 605 million in 2000 to 1.2 billion by the year 2025 (UN 1999). In 2000, for the first time, there will be more people aged 60 and older than children under 14 in a number of developed countries (UN 1999). Population ageing could be compared to a silent revolution that will impact on all aspects of society. It is imperative to prepare ourselves

The presentation made in Berlin on the occasion of Professor Egon Diczfalusy's 80th birthday celebrations was largely based on an article published in the journal *Science Progress Millennium Issues of the Year 2000* under the title "The Greying World: A Challenge for 21st Century".

in the most appropriate way for it: the opportunities and the challenges are multiple.

1.1 The Demographic Transition

The process of population ageing is driven by two major factors: increased life expectancy and declining fertility rates. This process is commonly referred to as the "demographic transition".

It is often assumed that most of the aged population live in developed countries. The reverse is true. Currently around 60% of the aged live in developing countries. Furthermore, those countries will be experiencing the steepest increase in the older population segment within the foreseeable future. In China, for example, the population 60 years and older will increase from 128 million in 2000 to 288 million in 2025 – that is, a larger elderly population than the total USA population today. Respective figures for Brazil are 13 and 32 million and for Nigeria 5.5 and 10 million: doubling of the older population in only 25 years. In other countries, such as Indonesia, Colombia, Kenya and Thailand, increases will be even higher – between 300 and 400 percent – i.e. up to 8 times higher than the increases, within the same period, in already aged societies such as Western European countries, where population ageing

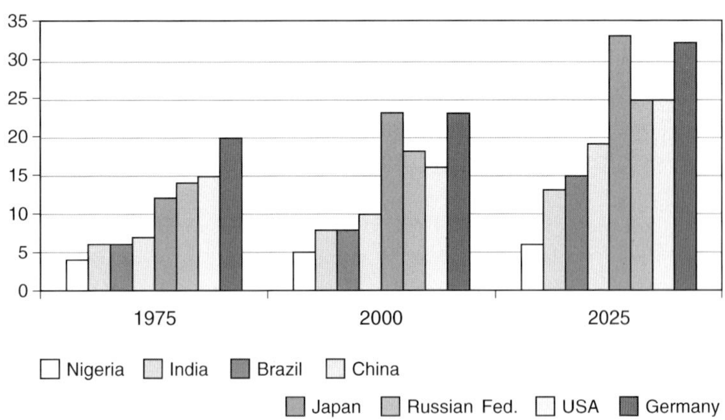

Fig. 1. Population 60 years and over as percentage of total population in selected countries in 1975, 2000 and 2025

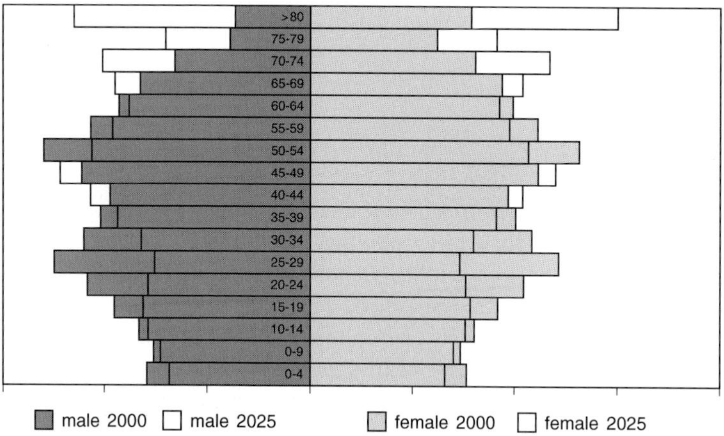

Fig. 2. Population pyramid for Japan in 2000 and 2050

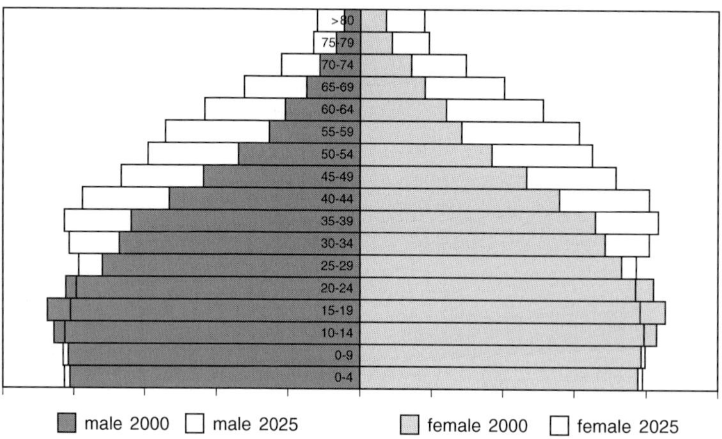

Fig. 3. Population pyramid for Brazil in 2000 and 2050

occurred over a much longer period of time. For example, it took 114 years in France for the aged population to increase from 7% to 14% (from 1865 to 1979), and 82 years in Sweden (from 1890 to 1972) (JARC 1998). The same doubling will occur in China in less than 30 years from 2000 to 2027 (US Department of Commerce 1993).

In addition to the increases in absolute numbers, important increases in the proportions of older people within the general population are expected in virtually all countries of the world the exception being in the Sub-Saharan region as indicated by the example of Nigeria in Fig. 1. By the year 2025 Italy will be the "oldest country" with 34% of its population aged 60 years or over, followed by Japan (32%) and Germany (31%). Throughout the world women outnumber men in old age.

Figures 2 and 3 show the population pyramids for Japan and Brazil summarising ageing trends worldwide in the first decades of the twenty-first century. Brazil will experience a steady decline in the proportions of youth and children while Japan's population structure will show further and substantial ageing of its population.

Figure 4 shows life expectancy at birth for men and women in selected countries. As a reflection of worldwide trends, in all of the selected five countries substantial increases in life expectancy at birth for both sexes have been registered over recent years and are likely to continue. Except for India in 1975, women expect to outlive men in all these countries for the selected years.

In most of the world fertility rates have experienced important declines over the last 25 years and by 2025 most countries will show total fertility rates[1] close to or below replacement-level[2] in most countries. Examples are given in Table 1. By 2025, only in Nigeria will total fertility rates be higher than replacement level. Indeed, it is estimated that already by 2010, 89 countries will have reached or will have rates below the 2.1 replacement level, a substantial increase compared to 1975, when just 26 countries had a total fertility rate below or equal to the replacement level (UN 1999).

The demographic transition can clearly be illustrated by the following data from Chile. Only 63% of the children born in 1909 reached their fifth birthday and only 13% of this birth cohort are living beyond the 85th birthday. In comparison, of the 1999 cohort only 2% will have died before their 5th birthday, and virtually half are expected to live beyond their 85th birthday (WHO 1999a).

---

[1] Definition: the average number of births each woman between 15 and 49 years would have if her lifetime fertility equalled the fertility of women of successive ages measured at the same time (WHO 1996).

[2] Replacement-level fertility is the total fertility rate of 2.1 children per woman.

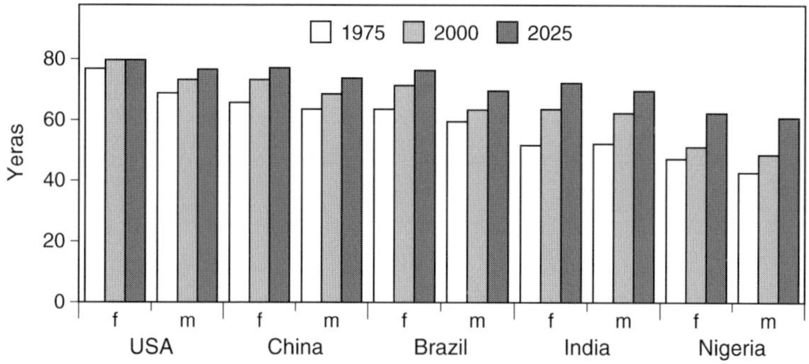

Fig. 4. Life expectancy at birth for women and men in selected countries in 1975, 2000 and 2025. (*f*), female; (*m*), male

Table 1. Total fertility rate in selected countries in 1975, 2000 and 2025

Country	Years 1975	2000	2025
Germany	1.5	1.3	1.6
USA	1.8	1.9	1.9
Japan	1.8	1.5	1.7
Russian Fed.	1.9	1.4	1.7
China	3.3	1.8	1.9
Brazil	4.3	2.1	2.1
India	4.8	2.7	2.1
Nigeria	6.9	4.7	2.7
Pakistan	7	4.5	2.1

Source: UN 1998.

With increasing numbers of older persons, the ratio between the aged and the working age population (15–64 years) will be increasing. This is shown for selected countries in Fig. 5. The ratio will virtually double in the USA, the Russian Federation, China and Brazil. In Nigeria, as an illustration of sub-Saharan Africa in general – the ratio will remain lowest among the selected countries.

Japan, one of the oldest countries in the world and the one currently enjoying the highest life expectancy at birth, will experience a threefold increase in the old-age dependency ratio between 1975 and 2025. While

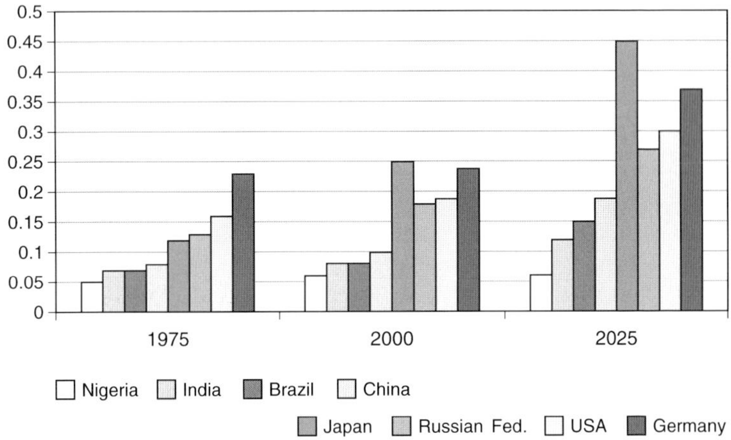

Fig. 5. Old age dependency ratio in selected countries. Old age dependency ratio is the quotient of the number of people age 65 and over by the number of people between 15 and 64 years (working age population). Source: UN 1999

in the mid-1960s 11 persons of working age were counted per one old adult (more precisely, a ratio of 8.5%), in 1996 there were only five persons of the working age population supporting one old adult (more precisely, a ratio of 21.8%). This figure is projected to increase to 59.1% in 2050 – i.e. for every two Japanese persons of working age, there will be one old person age 65 or older (JARC 1998).

2 Consequences of Ageing

2.1 The Epidemiological Transition

Population ageing will increasingly bring important challenges to health-care policymakers. This is particular so considering the changing pattern of diseases, translated into changing causes of death and morbidity – commonly referred to as the "epidemiological transition". The term "epidemiological transition" describes the increasing importance of disease and death attributable to non-communicable diseases (NCD) while those caused by infectious diseases decrease. The "epidemiological transition" has already been observed in virtually all developed countries and is now taking place in most of the developing world. For example, data from a sample cohort born in Chile 1909 show that the main causes of deaths were respiratory infections (20%), other infectious diseases (13%) and cardiovascular diseases (12%) – whereas cardiovascular diseases (31%) and cancers (23%) estimated were the major causes of death for Chileans in 1999 (WHO 1999a). While obviously welcome, the shift away from infectious diseases towards NCD will pose a different sort of challenge for developing countries. In 1990 about 40% of all deaths in developing countries were attributable to communicable diseases, around 50% to NCD, the remaining attributable to external causes of death (mostly accidents). By 2020, a very different picture will have emerged and NCD may be responsible for over 3/4 of the deaths in developing countries, according to WHO estimates. That is not to say, however, that infectious diseases will have disappeared in the foreseeable future, although they are expected to decrease in their importance as cause of morbidity. Either for their treatment or for their prevention, resources will continue to be required. At the same time, NCD will increase in both prevalence and cause of death in most of the developing world. The term "double burden of disease" has been used to reflect what could be the dominant nature of public health within the next few decades for the majority of developing countries.

2.2 The Challenge for Health Systems

With increasing proportions of older persons in the population, the demands to health care systems in developing countries will gradually change. Health care systems will be expected to accommodate care of older adults alongside, for example, child and maternal care. Since health systems are currently based on providing care to acute episodic conditions, they are not geared towards chronic-care needs and especially care for the aged. In particular, policymakers will be increasingly required to give emphasis to the degree of preparedness of the primary health sector to meet the demands created by population ageing – i.e. away from an exclusive focus on acute episodes towards the provision of chronic care in the community of conditions that cannot be cured and require continuing monitoring. More advanced health care systems in

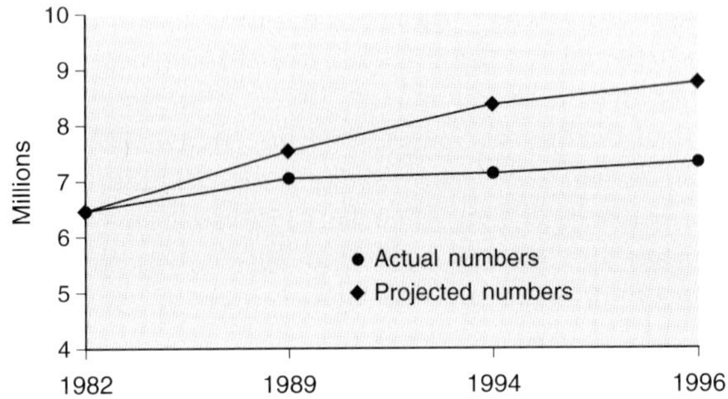

Fig. 6. Chronically disabled Americans 65 years and older. Source: US LTC Survey 1997

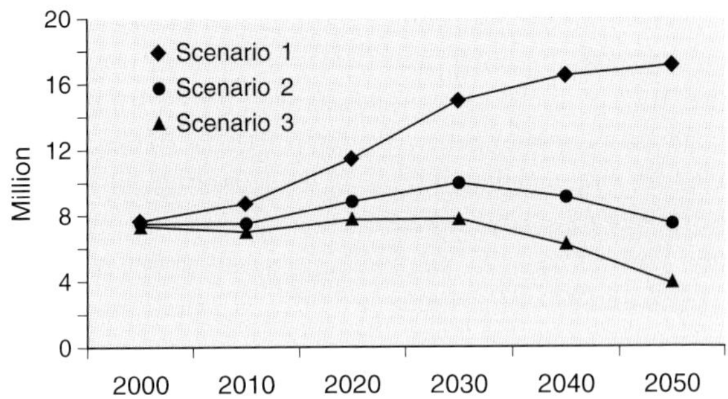

Fig. 7. Projections of disabled population aged 65+ years using 0% (Scenario 1), 1.1% (Scenario 2), and 1.5% (Scenario 3) annual decease

the developed world will also have to adapt to the shifting needs due to further population ageing. This does not imply that ageing is in itself a disease and old age should not be seen as equal to frailty, sickness and a high demand of health care services. Recent evidence coming from developed countries is encouraging. As data from the US Long Term Care Survey (1997) in Fig. 6 show, the disability rates of people aged 65 and over in 1996 were considerably lower than predicted. The rate of decline is impressive. If maintained or increased, the total numbers of disabled elderly people in the USA within the next few decades may stabilise or even diminish as seen in Fig. 7 (WHO, own calculations), if recent trends of decreasing age-related disability continue.

In the literature, discussions on how ageing influences health care expenditure have received increasing attention particularly since the mid-1960s. The main focus of such discussions centres around health care expenditures for acute health care. In 1980, Fries published the "compression of morbidity" hypothesis, suggesting that chronic disease would occupy only a small part of the entire life span – "compressed" into the very end of life while life expectancy would continue to rise to a set, biological limit of around 85 years. According to Fries' hypothesis, the number of very old persons would not increase beyond such limit and the period of physical disability would decrease, mainly due to improved public health measures and health promotion translated into lifestyle changes. While some of his views were subsequently challenged, a series of recent studies on health care expenditures in old age seem to support his hypothesis of the "compression of morbidity" (McCall 1984; Spector and Mor 1984; Riley et al. 1987; Roos et al. 1987; Temkin-Greener et al. 1992; Lubitz and Riley 1993; Busse et al. 1996; Zweifel et al. 1996). Several authors relate the higher acute health care expenditures/acute health service utilisation in old age not to age per se, but to the closeness to death ("the high costs of dying", Ginzberg 1980, supported by Fuchs 1984; i.e. rising costs are related to care close to death independent of an individuals' age). This hypothesis is also supported by recent data from a study using German sickness fund data, showing that hospital utilisation (per year) is related to age at time of death rather than age per se (Busse et al. 1996). Another study analysing data from a Swiss sickness fund also supported this hypothesis; the data showed that the health care expenditures in the last quarter of the last year of life were 300% higher than in the first quarter of the last year of life in a cohort of persons age 65 and over at the time of death (Zweifel et al. 1996). An interesting perspective is provided by an analysis of Medicare[3] (not covering nursing home costs) expenditures in the USA. The study showed that Medicare costs decline with increasing age at death. This may indicate that the very old (80 years and over) are not treated with highest technology available, rather with palliative care.

---

[3] Medicare is the public insurance program covering certain health care expenditures of the aged (65 and over), the permanently disabled and people with end-stage renal disease in the US Medicare is the single largest payer in the US medical care system and is financed through mandatory payroll taxes and premiums paid by the aged (Iglehart 1992).

Another recent study from Germany (Breyer 1999) indicated that the contribution of advances in medical care to the increased health care expenditures is highly underestimated, whereas the contribution of population ageing is being overestimated. The author suggested that factors which influence provider-driven demand and prescribing practices, as well as availability and access to services, should be taken into account when analysing health care expenditures. He concluded that ageing is not the only factor (maybe even one of the smallest factors) which affects the rising health care expenditures in the developed world.

Population ageing also modifies the demand for informal and formal long-term care. Although worldwide the bulk of care for frail elderly people is still provided by the family – particularly by an older female member of the family – changes in family structure and increasing participation of women in the paid work force are gradually eroding the capacity of the family to provide care (WHO/Milbank Memorial Fund 2000). Accordingly, new models of home care, provided by professionals to support the family, but avoiding costly stays in nursing home are being explored in most developed countries.

In the developing world, where health care systems are struggling with the double burden of diseases, the issues are even more complex. There is a strong need for training primary health care personnel in prevention and treatment of non-communicable diseases as well as for adapting health care systems in order to prepare them for an aged population. This is particularly important in areas where no health insurance or pension schemes exist. New and innovative schemes of community health care and long term care for the aged are urgently required to counteract factors such as disrupted family ties due to, for example, the trend towards nuclear families, migration to cities of young people, increasing participation of women in the paid labour force and, particularly in sub-Saharan Africa, the HIV/AIDS epidemics leaving orphaned children to be looked after by their grandparents. Above all, "a society for all ages" – the slogan adopted by the United Nations for the International Year of Older Persons celebrated in 1999 – has to be built on the foundations of a culture of solidarity – between generations, between different sectors and between nations.

2.3 Socioeconomic Consequences

Where available, public and private pension schemes are major contributors for protecting old people from poverty. Most of these schemes are still restricted to the developed world, but the number of countries implementing pension schemes is growing. Traditionally, funding resources for post-retirement come from three sources: a compulsory state pension, a (supplementary) occupational pension and individual savings. A forth source is gradually emerging: a combination of public pension and continued (part-time) work – as trends in some Western countries indicate (Geneva Association 1997). These continuing work schemes take advantage of the fact that many older employees have a higher ability to, for example, conduct meetings, handle persons diplomatically or see a problem before it emerges (The Economist 1999).

The future financing of pension schemes places economic challenges on virtually all countries even when considering the most optimistic forecasts. By and large, pension schemes were set up at times of low unemployment and low dependency ratios. With changes in age and employment structures, there is an urgent need for adaptation in these systems. In this respect, it is particularly important to note that life expectancy in old age has experienced substantial increases over recent decades. For example, 5.9 years for women aged 65 from 1960 to 1990 in Japan, 4.3 in France and 3.1 in the USA in the same 30 years [Organisation for Economic Co-operation and Development (OECD)

Table 2. Life expectancy at age 65 in selected countries

Country	Women 1996	Women 1986	Men 1996	Men 1986
Japan	25.9	23.6	20.8	19.7
France	25	23.2	19.7	18.1
Canada	24.3	23.2	19.9	18.4
Sweden	24	22.9	20	18.5
Australia	23.8	22.6	19.6	18.2
Greece	22.9	21.2	19.9	18.2
USA	22.9	22.4	19.2	17.9
Mexico	22.6	21.2	19.1	18.2
Poland	20.5	19.7	15.8	15.3
Hungary	19.4	18.6	14.9	14.6

Source: OECD, Health Data 1998.

Health Data 1998]. These increases have persisted more recently as shown in Table 2. To be noted is not only the substantial increases (of more than 2 years for women in Japan for instance) but that in relatively poor OECD countries – such as Greece and Mexico – life expectancy in old age is the same if not higher than in much richer countries such as the USA.

Most Western countries have been undertaking substantial reforms in their public pension systems, especially taking into consideration that the "baby-boom" generations are now approaching retirement age. Main features of these reforms are:

- The increase of retirement age. For example, in 1983, in the USA, it was agreed to gradually increase retirement age from 65 to 67 years within the period 2001–2027. Further, in Japan retirement age will be raised from 60 to 65 years between 2001 and 2013, and in Germany retirement age was set to 65 years.
- Increasing flexibility of retirement age and promotion of gradual retirement. Belgium was the first European country to introduce such a scheme, where retirement can be flexible between 60 and 65 years of age.
- Increased contribution period and freedom to combine pension with work income. The number of contribution years was recently increased in several European countries – from 37.5 to 40 years. The combination of limited work income in addition to the public pension is now possible in all EU countries. This is one of the newest characteristics of public pension schemes: (part-time) work continues for some years after the "official" retirement age, thus wage and public pension supplement each other. This system makes a significant contribution to reducing the constraints on publicly financed pension schemes. Also in the US, recent changes in policy such as the prohibition of a set retirement age by a company, or raising additional benefits an employee can accumulate through delaying retirement age have removed some barriers discouraging employment of older workers (The Economist 1999). Benefits for employers (e.g. reduced wage-cost per hour and decreased overall absenteeism – attributed to older workers "setting the example") and employees (e.g. adaptation of work to abilities in older age, benefits of staying longer as a member of the paid work force; extended possibilities for

professional contacts) are observed where such schemes have been implemented.

- Curtailing early retirement as a mediating feature between programmes to decrease occupational life and social policies to increase retirement age. Employees will not necessarily leave work earlier, but the costs of early retirement are then borne by the individual or the firm and not the state anymore. In France and Germany, such a feature is visible in current reforms, where costs are shared between the state, the employer and the employee.
- Reduced level of pension benefits. This was, for example, introduced in Denmark through taxation of pensions and through linking pension to price not to wage, as adopted by France, Sweden, Portugal and the United Kingdom.
- Changing the funding of public pension schemes, so that it depends less on contributions and more on taxes, as the examples of Sweden, Spain and Finland show. The advantage of such schemes is a reduction of costs of labour at a time of high unemployment (Geneva Association 1997).

In most developing countries "retirement age" is mostly non-existent for the majority of the population. The aged continue to work in small-scale farming, the informal sector or artisan undertakings, where they frequently play a crucial role in teaching their skills to younger generations, ensuring them employment opportunities. Old persons becoming too frail to work largely rely on their family to be cared for, especially daughters or daughters-in-law (Hoskins 1993).

While population ageing is certainly a challenge for health care and social security systems in developed countries, developing countries remain largely unprepared for the ageing of their populations. For the rich world, it could be said that the prospects of ageing have never been so good. Resources are in place and provided that there is political will, future cohorts of older people will benefit from unprecedented developments in medical technology to deal with ageing-associated diseases – coupled with the economic basis to provide them with renewed opportunities for leisure, education and social benefits. The same does not apply to the developing world. In essence, industrialised countries became rich before they became old, while developing countries will become old before they become rich.

3 Issues to Be Considered on Ageing and Health

3.1 Gender and Ageing

It is commonly assumed that "men and women age the same way", while in reality differences in the process of ageing vary greatly according to gender – hence a gender perspective on ageing is indispensable. In the vast majority of countries, women live longer than men do. Typically the difference is between 5 and 8 years; for instance, in countries like France and Brazil, women live about 8 years longer than men and about 6 years in Japan and the USA (UN 1999). However, there are exceptions such as in Eastern Europe, where the female advantage is as high as 12 years (e.g. Russian Federation, Latvia) while in Bangladesh and Kuwait there is virtually no difference.

Part of women's advantage with respect to life expectancy is biological; other explanatory factors are lifestyle and socioeconomic issues. There is, as yet, no complete understanding of why women outlive men and various hypotheses have been advanced. It is observed, for example, that an excess male mortality exists in the first 6 months of life. This "robustness" of baby girls may be attributed to varying chromosomal structure, but further investigation is needed. In adult life endogenous hormones protect women from ischaemic heart disease until menopause.

In contrast with such longer life expectancy at birth – and at subsequent stages of life – in studies on subjective morbidity and/or health perceptions, women frequently report more health problems than men. Women are more likely to suffer from ageing-related chronic diseases such as hypertension, diabetes, osteoporosis, arthritis or incontinence, which often result in reduced quality of live (WHO 1998). For example, the death rate (per 100,000 population, all ages) for musculoskeletal diseases was 3.5 for men and 10.0 for women in the United Kingdom in 1996. Respective figures for Germany are 1.6 and 3.9 and for the US, 1.9 and 4.7 (1994) (WHO 1996). Also in terms of burden of disease, measured by DALYs (disability adjusted life years), musculoskeletal diseases contributed in 1998 to 1.1% of the DALYs for men, but 2.1% for women, globally (WHO 1999a). Furthermore, as women age they are increasingly affected by coronary heart diseases – still erroneously perceived as "male" conditions. In 1998, 34% of all female deaths worldwide were attributable to cardiovascular diseases, compared to 28% in men (WHO 1999a). In Europe, for example, more than half of all women over 75 experience some form of disability due to heart disease (European Institute of Women's Health 1996).

With increasing economic development and social welfare, several traditional hazards to women's health are gradually being removed, particularly in terms of reproductive health. For instance, in Western European countries the life expectancy gender gap increases with socio-economic development (WHO 1998). As a result, in the oldest old age groups women predominate and are expected by 2025 to account for 2/3 of those aged 80 and over in countries such as France, Japan and Brazil and the USA (UN 1999).

However, the life-expectancy-at-birth gap between men and women in many countries is decreasing because of increased risk factors for chronic disease in women. A gender perspective on ageing and health should not, of course, be restricted to women. The health aspects of ageing men should not be neglected: "There is an urgent need to obtain...information on men" stated the Weimar Initiative "Healthy Aging for Men" (The International Society for the Study of the Aging Male 1998). In addition to biological factors, there are socioeconomic and health determinants that help to explain why women outlive men. For example, men are more often exposed to occupational hazards, have higher rates of accidents, drink alcohol more excessively and tend to smoke more (even tough in recent years a changing pattern is visible: women increasingly smoke, especially in developing countries). Furthermore, in most cultures men are made to believe that they are "undestroyable", hence hardly in need for medical attention (Kalache 1998). Often the only contacts occur in childhood before men return to medical attention in later life when it may be too late for preventive measures for conditions such as coronary heart diseases or for early detection of diseases such as cancers (Stückelberger, A., quoted in Kalache 1998).

3.2 Contributions of Older Persons

A common misconception associated with ageing relates to the participation and contributions made by older people to society. So often it is argued that "older people have nothing to contribute and are an economic burden to society". In reality, older persons make innumerable contributions to their families, their communities and to societies at large. Substantial contributions are made, for instance, within the informal sector and the unpaid labour force or as volunteers (as carers, community leaders or by teaching). In the United States, for example, there are over 3 million persons aged 65 and over actively involved in volunteer activities in health and political organisations, schools and religious organisations – in addition to many more millions of older persons providing "informal" care in the community (WHO 1999d). All these contributions to society remain (mostly) neglected in national macroeconomic indicators. The group contributing the most are older women, through their significant role as carers for their spouses and grandchildren. The universal trend towards more younger women joining the paid work force – a reflection of their higher educational levels together with the need to supplement the family income – makes older women indispensable as family caregivers and community workers throughout the world.

The extent to which older persons are involved in the care sector is illustrated by their role within the context of the AIDS epidemics in Africa.

3.2.1 Case Study: AIDS in Africa and Older Carers

Out of the 34 countries hardest hit by HIV and AIDS, 29 are in sub-Saharan Africa, three in Asia and two in Latin American and the Caribbean (UN 1999). In these countries the spread of AIDS/HIV infection is devastating the adult population, leaving their orphaned children behind. A recent study from southwest Uganda shows that 10% of the children under 15 years of age had lost both parents (Kamali et al. 1996). In other countries the situation is even gloomier. For instance in Zimbabwe, one in every five adults is infected (UN 1999) leading to the prospect of 18% of its children becoming orphans by 2010 (Kamali et al. 1996). For the same year, a predicted 17% of all children in Botswana and 12% in Tanzania will be orphans due to AIDS, most of them to be raised, nourished and educated by their grandparents (UNDP 1998). It is estimated that there will be 16 million children orphaned by AIDS in Africa by 2015 (Rutayuga 1992).

This is a critical developmental issue for African and other similarly HIV-affected developing countries, with significant implications for future human capital. The trauma of losing one or both parents is often magnified by relocation, possibly from an urban to a rural living environment, within the extended family structure. The burden of care and support falls mostly on only slightly older brothers and sisters and on the grandparents (Drew et al. 1998). A clash of generations often ensues. This may result in children or young adults straying from the family, ending up at higher risk for HIV infection, and then perpetuating the cycle of the disease. Information and support for those older people providing care is essential to prevent an overextension of family capacities to care for family members with AIDS, and subsequently to care for their orphaned children (Kamali et al. 1996; Seely et al. 1993).

These particularly affected countries need additional information and assistance in establishing support systems for older population forced to assume added roles as caregivers to their HIV-infected children and, subsequently, their grandchildren. WHO is now establishing firm collaboration with governmental agencies (UNAIDS) and the non-governmental organisation HelpAge International (HAI) to address the impact of this disease on older people in these countries. These projects will benefit from previous initiatives such as those examining grandparents caring for orphaned grandchildren in Zimbabwe and a survey in Thailand on health and socioeconomic needs of older persons and their families effected by the AIDS epidemic (Ageways 1996). More collaborative efforts like this will be necessary to define and assess the scope of the problem, the subsequent implications for older individuals, their extended families and society at large, and finally to strengthen the capacities of countries to develop solutions and policies to support this greatly affected older population.

Within the context of the active contributions older persons make to society, mainly through unpaid and voluntary work, it is important to consider the need for protecting and extending public pension and to provide paid work for those who need it. While there is no economic or biological basis for retiring at age 60 or 65, in countries dominated by the agricultural and informal, self-employment sectors, many older persons participate in the work force until they are physically unable to carry on and many would benefit from some respite well before then.

3.3 Urbanisation, Migration and Ageing

Urbanisation is another major recent global phenomenon. It is projected to continue well into the twenty-first century. While in 1980 close to 40% of the world's population were living in urban areas, it is now nearly 50% and projected to be 60% by 2020 (UN 1995). Urbanisation is a major reason behind the split of three-generation households. Together with migration between countries, urbanisation often leads to the need of grandparents acting as carers for their grandchildren left behind by their parents when they move to the city in search of employment. Most are unskilled workers and find it difficult to compete in the job market. Consequently, financial support to their families is usually low, leaving to the old relatives the difficult task of providing nourishment to themselves and their grandchildren. Care policies and care programmes on national and local levels need to reflect this global trend and include steps to support these aged carers, mainly women. All these issues will be carefully examined in the First Global Conference on Rural Ageing to take place in West Virginia in June 2000 (H. Hermanova, personal communication). The ageing process of previous migrants is often a particular challenge for individuals who have not fully been integrated into the "host" community, but who will feel particularly "up-rooted" once the changes common to ageing occur and the longing for more remote experiences becomes more acute.

In addition, urbanisation can also result in very frail older persons left isolated in rural areas as younger generations move to cities; as a consequence a disproportionate amount of aged persons are to be found among the poorest poor in rural settings. As social security schemes providing adequate pensions are rare, elderly persons left in rural areas often depend on financial support from their children living in the city – which may never reach them.

Adjustment to all these factors combined with loosening family values and erosion of cultural and traditional values is often difficult to older persons as they are themselves not being supported by their children in the same way they used to assist their own parents.

3.4 Functional Capacity and Ageing

"Older people are frail" is another common misconception related to ageing – as the reality is that the majority of older people remains physically fit well into old age. They continue to carry out activities for their daily living and therefore to play an active part in their community. In this respect, it is especially useful to exam the concept of functional capacity within a life course perspective as illustrated in Fig. 8.

Our capacity in relation to a number of functions (such as ventilatory capacity, muscular strength, cardiovascular output) increases in childhood and peaks in early adulthood. Such peak is eventually followed by a decline. How fast the decline progresses, however, is largely determined by factors related to adult lifestyle – such as smoking, alcohol consumption and diet. The natural decline in cardiac function, for example, can be accelerated by smoking, leaving the individual with a functional-capacity level lower than would normally be expected for his/her age. The gradient of decline may become so steep as to result in premature disability. However, the acceleration in decline may be reversible at any age. Smoking cessation and small increases in the level of physical

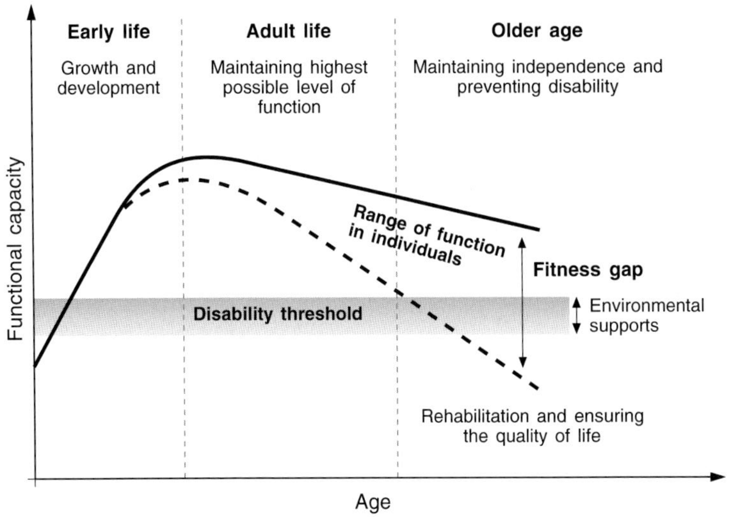

Fig. 8. A life-course perspective for maintenance of the highest possible level of functional capacity

Table 3. Action towards active ageing

Factors	Individual Action	Policy Action
Diet	Consume a diet high in fibre and low in animal fat and salt Reduce your body weight if you are overweight and maintain normal body weight	Increase consumer awareness about direct links between good nutrition and health
Physical activity	Exercise regularly from the earliest years through older ages	Incorporate exercise into school curricula Create workplaces which provide exercise facilities Encourage sports for seniors
Smoking	Stop smoking – cessation is beneficial at any age Educate children about the ill effects of smoking	Ban tobacco advertising Ban sale of tobacco to children Provide health education in schools and workplaces
Alcohol	Maintain moderate drinking habits Seek professional help if you think you may drink excessively	Ban sale of alcohol to children
Social integration	Stay involved in your family, your community, a club or religious organisation Be aware and speak out against ageism Continue to educate yourself and all your children	Support activities that foster social cohesion Provide access to life-long learning Promote solidarity among the generations

Source: WHO 1999d.

fitness, for example, reduce the risk of developing coronary heart disease.

In addition to these factor others, conditioned by social class, also affect functional capacity. Poor education, poverty, and harmful living and working conditions all make reduced functional capacity more likely in later life. In some countries, people with poor functional ability are more likely to become institutionalised, which in itself can lead to dependence, particularly for the small minority of older people who suffer from loss of mental function and/or confusion.

The slope of the decline can be influenced in any stage through individual as well as policy measures (see Table 3). For example, smoking cessation at age 50 reduces the risk of dying within the next 15 years by 50% (WHO 1999b).

For those who become disabled, provision of rehabilitation and adaptations of the physical environment can greatly reduce the level of disability. Furthermore, specific interventions can help them to improve their functional capacity and thus quality of life. For example, cataract, causing nearly 50% of all blindness worldwide, can be treated through a fairly simple surgical procedure, increasingly available in developing countries (WHO 1999c).

Quality of life should be a major consideration throughout the life-course, particularly for those whose functional capacity can no longer be maintained. For example, changes in the living environment can vastly improve quality of life. However, most of the gains are obtained by acting on the "care unit" – in most cases the family and close friends. It is often by supporting the informed carer (frequently an older woman, in many cases in poor health herself) that the quality of life of the dependent older person can be most improved.

Finally, through appropriate environmental changes – such as adequate public transportation in urban environments, the availability of lifts in apartment or office blocks, ramps, adapted kitchenware or a toilet seat with rails – the disability threshold can be lowered. Such changes can ensure a more independent life well into very old age, and one of the major challenges is to ensure access to them to all older persons – including the poor and those who live in remote areas.

Encapsulating the "functional capacity" approach, the World Health Organization Ageing and Health Programme has developed an "active ageing" conceptual framework. Active ageing can be defined as "the process of optimising opportunities for physical, social, mental and economic well-being throughout the life course in order to extend healthy life expectancy". (Ministry of Health, Canada 1999) This process can be instrumental for the global challenge of ensuring that individuals grow older in good health and actively participate in society.

4 Facing the Challenge: The WHO Ageing and Health Programme (Now Ageing and Life Course, ALC) and Its Partners

In April 1995 the World Health Organization launched the Ageing and Health Programme, replacing the former Health of the Elderly Programme. In developing its response to global ageing, AHE has incorporated the following perspectives:

- A life course perspective of ageing rather than compartmentalising the health care of "the elderly"
- Health promotion, focusing on active ageing – physically, socially and mentally, since whether early or later in life, people have multiple opportunities to improve their health status as they age, provided they are properly supported by the environment (physical and social) where they live
- A socioeconomic, cultural and an ethical perspective, paying tribute to the fact that the settings where individuals age play an important part in their health and well-being
- A gender perspective – recognising the important differences in men's and women's health and way of life, which become more pronounced in later life
- An intergenerational perspective – emphasising strategies to maintain cohesion between the generations
- An ethical perspective – enhancing the understanding of ethical issues such as human rights, elder abuse, long-term care as well as undue prolongation or hastening of death
- A community-oriented perspective, since throughout the world, even in the rich societies, the majority of older persons live in the community and most of their problems will have to be dealt with at the community level

ALC activities are concentrated into four major programme components: information dissemination, capacity building through research and training, advocacy, and policy development. Each of the programme components incorporates the programme perspectives mentioned before. Through the development of these four programme components

ALC expects a global strategy on active ageing to become increasingly focused and effective.

Since 1999, the last year of the twentieth century, was designated by the United Nations as the "International Years of Older Persons" under the theme "A Society for All Ages", AHE has used the opportunity to enhance its advocacy role. A special effort was made to create a stable network of people (policy makers, researchers, activists, NGOs and governmental officers) interested in working towards common active ageing policies on national and international level. This "Global Movement for Active Ageing" network was launched on 2 October[4] 1999 through a global walk event. In every time zone of the globe, several cities organised a walk event for and with the aged. The events included intergenerational celebrations, festivals for health promotion, exercise through walking, traditional dancing and other sports, as well as celebrations of culture, traditions and wisdom, which the aged can share with the other generations. There were over 2,000 cities in more than 90 countries from all five continents involved. This "Global Embrace" was successfully repeated on 1 October 2000 – again with a massive response to WHO call around the world. The "Global Movement for Active Ageing"[5] will continue to expand as a network for information exchange, mutual support and policy formulation well into the next century.

The international community has not yet fully demonstrated an awareness to population ageing through firm action. The response is still patchy and weak. Perhaps the opportunity of the Second UN Assembly on Ageing – to take place in April 2002 in Madrid, Spain – will be the call to nations that the twenty-first century will be characterised by global ageing. History will judge if we – collectively – will have demonstrated the resolve to face the challenges ahead of us. If we fail, we will be our own victims: adults today, tomorrow's older citizens.

---

[4] The 1 October is celebrated every year as the International Day of Older Persons. Since the 2 October 1999 is a Saturday, this day was chosen for organisational reasons.

[5] For further information please visit the web page www.who.int/hpr/ageing or e-mail activeageing@who.ch

References

Ageways 40 (1996) Newsletter. HelpAge International, London, April:11–12

Breyer F (1999) Private and public choices in health and health care. Paper prepared for the 2nd World Conference of the iHEA (June), Rotterdam

Busse R, Schwartz FW, Schulenburg M von der, et al (1996) Leistungen und Kosten der medizinischen Versorgung im letzten Lebensjahr, Norddeutscher Forschungsverbund Public Health – Projekt D3, Abschlußbericht, Hannover

Drew RS, Makufa C, Foster G (1998) Strategies for providing care and support to children orphaned by AIDS. AIDS Care 10 [Suppl 1]:S9–S11

European Institute of Women's Health (1996) Women in Europe towards healthy ageing. A review of the health status of mid-life and older women, Dublin

Fries JF (1980) Aging, natural death, and the compression of morbidity. N Engl J Med 303(3):130–135

Fuchs VR (1984) "Though much is taken": reflections on aging, health, and medical care. Milbank Mem Fund Q Health Soc 62:143–166

Geneva Association (1997) The future of retirement in Europe, a summary of recent reforms of public (1st pillar) pensions, research programme on social security, insurance and saving and employment, 21bis, Geneva, July

Ginzberg E (1980) The high cost of dying. Inquiry 17:293–295

Hoskins I (1993) Combining work and care for the aged: an overview of the issues. Int Labour Rev 123(3):347

Iglehart JK (1992) The American health system – Medicare. N Engl J Med 327:1467–1472

International Society for the Study of the Aging Male (1998) The Weimar initiative, appendix. Aging Male Vol 1 1:7

Japan Aging Research Centre (1998) Aging in Japan 1998, Tokyo

Kalache A (1998) Health and the ageing male, World Health, 51st year. 5:Sept–Oct

Kamali A, Seely JA, Nunn AJ, Kengeya-Kayondo JF, Ruberantwari A, Mulder DW (1996) The orphan problem: experience of a sub-Saharan Africa rural population in the AIDS epidemic. AIDS Care 8(5):509–515

Lubitz JD, Riley GF (1993) Trends in Medicare payments in the last year of life. N Engl J Med 328:1092–1096

McCall N (1984) Utilization and costs of Medicare services by beneficiaries in their last year of life. Med Care 22:329–342

Ministry of Health, Canada (1999) Oral communication

Murray C, Lopez A (1996) The global burden of disease. Harvard University Press

OECD (1998) Health Data, databank

Riley G, Lubitz J, Prihoda R, Rabey E (1987) The use and costs of Medicare services by cause of death. Inquiry 24:233–244

Roos NP, Montgomery P, Roos LL (1987) Health care utilization in the years prior to death. Milbank Q 65:231–254

Rutayuga JB (1992) Assistance to AIDS orphans within family/kinship system and local institution: a program for East Africa, AIDS Educ Prev [Fall Suppl]:57–58

Seely J, Kajura E, Bachengana C, Okongo M, Wagner U, Mulder D (1993) The extended family and support for people with AIDS in a rural population in southwest Uganda: a safety net with holes? AIDS Care 5(1):117–122

Spector WD, Mor V (1984) Utilization and charges for terminal cancer patients in Rhode Island. Inquiry 21:328–337

Temkin-Greener H, Meiners MR, Petty EA, Szydlowski JS (1992) The use and cost of health services prior to death: a comparison of the Medicare-only and the Medicare-Medicaid elderly populations. Milbank Q 70:679–701

The Economist (1999) Ageing workers – a full life. Sept 4, pp 75ff

United Nations (1999) World population prospects. The 1998 Revision

United Nations (1995) Population database

UNDP (1998) Human development report 1998. Oxford University Press, New York

US Department of Commerce (1993) An aging world II, international population reports P95/92–3. Washington D.C.

US Long Term Care Survey (1996) http://www.cds.duke.edu/NLTCS_INTRO:html

WHO (1996) World Health Statistics

WHO (1998) Gender and health, WHO/FRH/WHD/98.16, Geneva

WHO (1999a) World Health Report 1999, Geneva

WHO (1999b) AHE; fact sheet on ageing and tobacco. Published for World Health Day 1999b. Available on request from AHE through activeageing@who.ch

WHO (1999c) AHE; Fact sheet on ageing and visual disability, published for World Health Day 1999c. Available on request from AHE through activeageing@who.ch

WHO (1999d) Ageing – exploding the myths, WHO/HSC/AHE/99.1. Geneva

WHO/MMF (2000) Towards an international consensus on policy for long-term care of the ageing, WHO/HSC/AHE/00.1, Geneva

World Bank (1998) World development indicators

Zweifel P, Felder S, Meier M (1996) Demographische Alterung und Gesundheitskosten: Eine Fehlinterpretation. In: Oberender P (ed) Alter und Gesundheit. Gesundheitsökonomische Beiträge 26. Nomos, Baden-Baden, pp 29–46

3 The Challenge for the Pharmaceutical Industry

G. Stock

1 Introduction

Our health care system is facing major challenges today and in the years to come – so is the pharmaceutical industry.

First of all, we are living in ageing societies, which means that the percentage of elderly people is increasing steadily. This has enormous consequences for health care systems and for health care costs in particular, since we all know that the need for medical care arises mainly in older age. Prevention of disability at old age, prevention and retardation of loss of function will be major tasks for the pharmaceutical industry. This also calls for early diagnosis and therapy in the case of a number of diseases with high incidence rates in the elderly population, like neurodegenerative diseases, especially Parkinson's and Alzheimer's diseases.

Secondly, since we are all affected by rigid cost containment in our health care systems, we will have to decide how to allocate or reallocate limited resources in order to be able to pay for innovative solutions. Cost-effectiveness is increasingly entering discussions and negotiations about reimbursement of drug costs but this does not provide the answer to the question how rising demands and expectations in the health care sector can be met in the future without killing innovation.

Thirdly, the results from research in genomics and molecular biology do not only hold out hope for significant progress in therapies but also the prospect of true innovations in the fields of diagnosis, prevention and treatment of hitherto untreatable diseases. New disciplines and technologies in drug research, like pharmacogenomics, proteomics, bioinformatics and high-throughput screening have completely changed our attitudes and approaches to drug discovery. Together with a growing understanding of the human genome and the functions and interactions of the proteins encoded by it, new and exciting possibilities to combat diseases will arise.

2 Demographics

As already mentioned, societies are getting older. The percentage of the elderly (people over 65 or even 75 years of age) will be increasing over the years to come. By 2050, there will be more people above the age of 65 in China than today's entire population of the United States, which is 270 million people. At present, about 5,000 people in the United States reach the age of 65 every day compared to 3,300 who die. What are the implications for the pharmaceutical industry? Whereas in the past our focus has been on age-dependent fatal chronic diseases, we will have to concentrate on preventive medicines and causal treatment of non-fatal age-dependent diseases like Alzheimer's disease and other neurodegenerative CNS conditions.

Prevention of disability or maintenance and restoration of functional capability, safeguarding the integrity and autonomy of the individual will be a major challenge of the future and a focus of our research activities. Of course this does not negate the ongoing need for innovation in oncology and cardiovascular diseases.

There is a difference in life expectancy between women and men. For example, in North America the average life expectancy of women is nearly 7 years greater than that of men, and in Europe the difference is even 8 years. It is our vision to reach a balance between the sexes in this respect, and Schering has responded to this challenge with a special research programme dedicated to the ageing male.

In summary, there is enormous room for innovation and there is also a real need for innovation in connection with the ageing society.

3 Cost Considerations

The dynamics of an ageing society together with the opportunities to develop new diagnostics and therapeutics offered by genomic research and molecular biology are major challenges for the pharmaceutical industry as well as for health care systems. With only 10%–20% of all known diseases today being causally treatable, the need for improved and for new therapeutic and diagnostic drugs is evident.

Health care spending has been fairly constant for the past few years amounting to about 7%–14% of the GDP, depending on the country. Pharmaceutical spending accounted for roughly 10%–15% of overall health care spending (exception: Japan).

It is obvious that these figures must rise in view of the demographics, the opportunities of modern medicine and the needs which I have just mentioned. But our society will not be able to pay for those new and innovative treatments unless it sets new priorities in the allocation of the total budget, a challenge which is closely connected with the question of how much our society will be prepared to spend for health.

Asking this question, we also have to consider the enormous economic benefits from new and effective drugs and treatments. We have to look at the direct costs avoided by the introduction of H_2-blockers in the case of peptic ulcers, for example, or of anticancer drugs in ALL (acute lymphocytic leukaemia), or oestrogen treatment to prevent hip fractures. We have to take into account the striking drop in death rates in early infancy diseases, rheumatic fever and rheumatic heart disease, atherosclerosis, to name but a few, due to new pharmaceuticals. And, last but not least, if we consider the dramatic decline in the average length of stay in hospitals, we get an idea of what the financial benefits of drugs, all too often ignored, amount to – drugs like nifedipine, captopril, gadolinium-DTPA or β-interferon – it is just a selection.

Rediscussing and re-evaluating the overall portfolio of public expenditure in the light of medical needs but also of new values defined by our society – like quality of life – will be a challenge which, however, offers new and attractive prospects not only for patients but also for our economy.

With a share of 10%–15% of overall health care costs, pharmaceuticals can hardly be blamed for being a cost driver, nor can the pharmaceutical industry. R&D expenditures are growing faster than the sales rates, which in fact have shown a slow-down in the past few years. In contrast, R&D costs have continually risen. In 1979 the average cost to bring a new chemical or biological entity to the market was 122 million euros. In 1999 it is nearly 5 times more, i.e. 560 million euros. This does not reflect bad management but more exacting demands with regard to efficacy, quality and safety. We have to spend more and more money for the innovation as such, but at the same time our development costs have risen tremendously, development costs to prove the efficacy in patients but also and for the much greater part to prove the safety of new drugs. In other words, the demand for money to demonstrate the innovation is creating a new requirement, namely to demonstrate the safety of this innovation. In today's thinking, this is quite natural and it seems to be obvious that we have to intensify our safety research. How big the hurdles of success before marketing authorization have become is shown by the fact that the number of new chemical entities reaching the market has constantly decreased since 1987 when it was 57, whereas in 1999 only 32 new chemical entities worldwide were introduced into the market. At the same time, the number of drugs in development has continuously increased amounting to more than 6,000 in 1999. This clearly shows that there is a trend from quantity to quality and also an obvious trend to higher failure rates during drug development.

According to a recent survey in the United States, R&D costs as percentage of sales increased from 11.9% in 1980 to an estimated 20.8% in 1999. Despite all our efforts to speed up drug development, it still takes 10 years and more on average from synthesis to drug approval and in addition, the time of market exclusivity for innovative drugs is steadily decreasing. The pharmaceutical industry is operating in a highly competitive environment and as new drugs are becoming more and more specific, patient numbers per drug will probably not increase but rather decrease. I do not believe that the number of blockbusters will dramatically increase; it will remain constant. By contrast, the number of drugs for specific patient populations will increase, and this development in our industry has its price.

If we look once more at the enormous spending in R&D, the question where all the money goes may reasonably be asked. Approximately 40% is spent on pre-clinical work, including drug research, another 40% on clinical work and then come process development, quality control and others. This, however, is a rather lump-sum kind of answer. As a matter of fact, we have to rethink radically how to spend our money in-house as well as externally. This is one of the major challenges ahead of us. How are we going to tackle the vast amount of new knowledge? How will we manage to master new technologies? Are we set for the future? Do our processes need re-engineering? Are there opportunities outside, like co-operations, to complement or bring synergies to our own expertise and skills? These and other questions are all challenges for the pharmaceutical industry that call for innovative approaches in research, development, infrastructure, life-cycle management and also in defensive measures. Innovation, which is an almost trivial term in itself, thus bears a lot of connotations in today's pharmaceutical industry. This brings me to another topic which largely escapes public awareness.

4 Paradigm Shift in Drug Research

We are a fairly young industry. In the 1950s, we had classical chemistry producing many, hundreds and thousands, of individual molecules which were all more-or-less innovative. The poor pharmacologist had somehow to cope with them and show some efficacy. There was a lot of blind-screening, of trial and error, of hit or miss. There was an almost unlimited number of possibilities, and the success rate was not too good.

Dramatic changes occurred in the 1960s, 1970s and 1980s. The pharmaceutical industry started rational drug finding, which means that in vitro testing, enzyme assays and receptor tests became the key elements of research. The chemist had to find different ligands and substrates for a limited number of targets: about 500 receptors and enzymes. Safety pharmacology was introduced in the 1970s, and in the 1980s the stage was set for a different scenario: proteins as drugs became fashionable, and the end of small-molecule chemistry was being predicted.

The 1990s marked another change which was dramatic in itself and had enormous consequences for research-based pharmaceutical industry. Almost all of a sudden we found ourselves in a completely different world. Genome research together with genomics and proteomics, combinatorial chemistry and high-capacity screening disclosed a virtually unlimited number of targets. There also was an unlimited number of tests to demonstrate efficacy at the molecular level. This has then to be translated into biological efficacy and the question arises: What does this mean for the organism as a whole? This is an enormous problem which has not been properly resolved, and we are just beginning to understand that the interplay of genes and proteins and their functions is far more complex than originally thought. But we have access to the genes, the cookbooks for the proteins, and we can modify the activity of the proteins with small molecules, which are back on the stage again and badly needed. New methods like gene therapy and gene diagnostics are opening a fantastic new world.

At the same time, patenting has become a complex issue. Formerly, it was enough to patent a chemical entity. Today, we try to patent genes and their functions, we try to patent proteins and their functions, and we try to patent respective ligands. This is close to impossible on one hand, in one institution or company, and we have to look for the different players in this field, the ones who know the gene, the ones who have the protein, the ones who know their functions. We have to find ways how to interact and co-operate with the different players. Thus patent strategy has become a highly important part of our R&D approaches.

Drug finding today is a whole world of different disciplines, and it is obvious that one cannot be the master of all of them in-house. A dramatic change, almost invisible for the outside, has therefore taken place within the past seven or eight years. For once, our company has been transformed from a research and development company into a research, search and development company. Search means looking for and establishing various levels of co-operation networks ranging from classical university-type institutions to small companies where we have access to new product ideas or to new technologies. And secondly, our researchers, besides their scientific capabilities, had to show that they are able to manage such networks. So a lot of mental change was required.

Our approach to meeting the challenges of today and the future can be described as a triangle whose corners constitute disease knowledge, enabling technologies and efficient partnership plus networking. These cornerstones provide the basis for innovation as a prerequisite for our leadership in specialized markets in the world.

To put all this into the right perspective, we should pause for a moment and consider some points that I think are particularly important:

- Genomics has revolutionized our working methods. Our way of thinking has been fundamentally changed by molecular medicine. Nevertheless, only a fraction of compound-finding projects in the pharmaceutical industry worldwide is completely and exclusively based on research in genomics. Targets that have been identified through research in genomics are thus still research objects today but not yet compound-finding objects. The future, in this respect, will be slower to enter our life than many prophets want us to believe.
- The amount of data emanating from future genome and protein research projects will become gigantic. Without meaningful and suitable linkages of these data, it will not be possible to adequately translate our accumulated knowledge into therapeutics and diagnostics.
- The multiplicity of genetic mutations and their detection will be a central element of future research.

5 Regulatory Issues

Time is money! This is especially true when it comes to the submission of our application for market authorization of a new drug. We have to go to regulatory authorities much earlier than we did in the past in order to discuss with them possible and acceptable endpoints of clinical studies, or toxicological, pharmacokinetic and other requirements, in short, ways to demonstrate the efficacy, quality and safety of a new drug. This will allow us to design and manage the development process in a way that saves time and money, for example by installing more parallel processes instead of sequential ones, by trying to avoid duplicating studies and so forth.

Formerly, dossiers comprised, more or less, a compilation of data and were submitted separately to individual country authorities. Nowadays, we have a process involving all major countries like Europe, Japan, the

United States. We are creating one global dossier meeting worldwide standards and requirements harmonized by regulatory authorities at an international level, which means that it is a high level. Thus, in 1988 when we submitted a dossier, this comprised about ten files full of paper. For the same compound today, we would have to submit about 30 files. On top of that, we now have to produce electronic files for those regulatory authorities who have the means to read them. It is a matter of logistics, and a costly one at that.

An additional issue has now gained utmost importance, that is the collection and reporting of side-effects on a world-wide scale. Within very tight time limits we have to report side-effects seen in any country of this world to health authorities in Europe, in USA, Japan and elsewhere, and we have to submit a full safety dossier to them at regular intervals. This requires a vast infrastructure and at the same time an enormous portion of professional behaviour.

The pharmaceutical industry is one of the most heavily regulated industries. We have people specialized in talking with authorities. Everything is regulated: chemical waste, animal experiments, gene technology, good manufacturing practice, clinical development and on and on. And there are inspections by regulatory authorities again and again.

It does not stop with the granting of a marketing authorization. When you are on the market you have to show what the product is really doing. Of course, all this costs money. We need more and new products and, therefore, we have to re-engineer development and approval processes.

6 The Future

I already mentioned some of the challenges that societies and the pharmaceutical industry in particular have to face today and in the future. Let me add another important issue which is changing our life more radically than we would have dared to dream only 2 or 3 years ago: the Internet and new media like the cellular phone. Both will have an enormous impact on the dialogue between industry, doctors, patients, patient groups as well as on their respective attitudes and behaviour. On the one hand, patients and patient groups will no longer faithfully accept and adhere to drugs and treatments prescribed by doctors. They will ask for options and turn to the Internet to make their own judgements.

Doctors will have to use pertinent databases to underpin their decisions. And pharmaceutical industry will increasingly have to perform outcomes research, a new discipline, to prove the benefits of its drugs. It will have to establish means to respond to the queries from both authorities and consumers. This is a growing issue both in terms of methodology and cost.

On the other hand, a confidence-building dialogue with patients through the Internet will become an essential element of our efforts to demonstrate our leadership in specialized markets.

And finally, electronic selling of pharmaceuticals will be an issue in the future, but we have not yet a clear picture how to tackle this.

I mentioned outcomes research, and this brings me to yet another issue that will have an enormous impact on our development process as well as on the chances of new drugs, and especially innovative ones, to gain regulatory approval. As I said, it is a young discipline that tries to analyse and put into relation all those factors and data that are relevant for determining the real value of drugs and health care interventions. It has to tussle with an enormously complex matter including aspects such as health outcomes, alternative treatment options, age, gender and other sociodemographic factors, length of disease, progression of disability, quality of life. Cost-effectiveness analyses are made to measure these aspects and their impact on costs. However, since different methodologies are employed, since different perspectives are adopted and since different objectives are envisaged, the outcome will be different. Whether you look at the direct medical costs only, or at the direct non-medical costs as well or consider indirect and intangible costs too, it will give you completely different pictures. The results of a burden of illness study cannot be compared with those of a cost-effectiveness analysis or a cost-utility analysis. Even when using the same methodology, you arrive at different results depending on the outcome measured, for example in multiple sclerosis (MS).

Increasingly, cost-effectiveness analyses are required as a precondition for reimbursement of drugs in a rising number of countries. However, effectiveness refers to a situation in real life, whereas the relatively artificial setting of clinical trials can essentially only provide efficacy data. Thus, pharmaceutical firms are required to provide data at the time of submission which can only be gathered after marketing authorization, during long-term use of a drug – outside clinical trials. Today's approach to calculating disease costs is in many cases a short-term (if not short-sighted) approach, looking at the cost per injection, the cost per hospital admission, the cost per drug treatment, etc. But many diseases like MS involve life-long medical and non-medical costs. Hence a period of time of say 20 or 30 years instead of 6, 9 or 12 months should be considered to arrive at a fair judgement of medical or medicinal interventions.

Sometimes it will be very difficult for a single drug to show its cost-effectiveness and it probably needs years to observe the field as such to see the cost benefit as can now be done after 30 years of drug treatment in heart disease, pneumonia or cerebrovascular diseases.

The more we learn about the natural history of diseases the more we will understand the need for frequent diagnostic procedures, the need for primary and secondary prevention and the need for intermittent and chronic treatment. Treatment, however, means more than drug treatment. Long-term patient observation and long-term cost considerations for a given disease will, therefore, gain greater importance in the future than today where we are still fiddling with a clear picture of acutely emerging costs in a given situation. Instead of snapshots, long-term follow-up will be increasingly demanded in order to come to a fair cost and cost-benefit judgement for a given patient.

How difficult, if not impossible, it can be to evaluate the true value of a drug can be shown with oral contraceptives. When Pinkus died, D.E. Cameron wrote in the *New York Times*: "Few contributions to medical knowledge have done so much to bring to women everywhere a sense of worth and dignity". How can we express this in terms of money?

We have to understand better the variables of cost-effectiveness studies, we have to establish the appropriate methodology and we have to enter into a dialogue with authorities to come to a common understanding of health outcomes, namely that it is a dynamic process involving incremental demonstration of value, which changes during a medicine's lifecycle.

This is a real challenge.

7 Schering's Answer to Challenges

How, then, will Schering meet all those challenges (there are quite a number of other important issues like knowledge management, bioinformatics, etc. that I have not mentioned)?

Our strategy for the future is built on a combination of detection, prevention and therapy. This means that in special fields we want to cover the whole spectrum of options to respond to the particular needs of diagnosis, of prophylaxis and of effective treatments. When I say special fields I am referring to areas that are not within the focus of major research and development efforts currently being pursued in the pharmaceutical industry. The big topics dealt with by the major pharmaceutical companies do not include fields like fertility control and hormone therapy. However, our company is still highly active also in these areas in which we have been engaged for quite some time, as you know. We stick to them because we believe that there is a future for them. Our approach will be different, though. For example, we no longer perceive women as different and separate age groups – girls, young, middle-aged, menopausal, climacteric and post-climacteric women. We rather look at them as females passing through different stages of their life, with changing needs and expectations regarding their health and well-being. So oral contraceptives are perfect for girls and young women who want to live their lives without fear of unwanted pregnancies. What about the middle-aged women? They have children and families but for various reasons they don't want to go back to the pill again. So we offer them a highly innovative intrauterine system, Mirena, to relieve them of their fear of unintentionally becoming pregnant at a time in their life when they do no longer feel fit for it. Then comes menopause, where we offer sequential hormone replacement therapy (HRT) to overcome the unpleasant accompanying circumstances. After that, the climacteric and the post-climacteric period warrants continuous HRT preparations. There will be a major breakthrough if we achieve what is badly needed, namely that women take HRT for longer than the usual 2 years. This is a major task for doctors, for the industry and for health professionals.

There will be active research on bone preservation, there will be active research on oncological topics, specifically for mammary, ovarian and all the endocrine-dependent tumours. At the same time, much educational work will have to be done to eliminate all the uncertainties and the ignorance regarding HRT both in doctors and their female patients. We can take over an important part in this respect but we need the help and support of institutions like WHO, with their credibility and their networks.

We deeply believe that the application of hormones in women at almost every stage of their life will have a benefit in terms of prevention of pregnancies, prevention of diseases, preservation of function. We are already offering a large variety of products to cover these fields. But with the existence of modern methods of genomics, of molecular biology and with new clinical research there will be major breakthroughs also in other fields than fertility control and hormone therapy and we are confident that female health care will offer a lot of opportunities for us. Thus, in summary, our strategy in this respect will be an integrated approach which, however, will also include the male as already mentioned. We call this approach gender-specific health care.

Now a final word, as a general remark to another type of challenge of the future. What does molecular medicine mean for countries that cannot spend so much money in the health care system such as the less developed countries? Does this new medicine offer chances or problems to those countries?

First of all, we have good examples how developed and less developed countries can co-operate in important fields such as fertility control. Here the non-profit organizations many years ago found agreements by which it became possible at low costs to provide all those countries with oral contraceptives, injectables and implants.

It would be worthwhile to think about similar programs in the field of HRT, which in an ageing society is a prime asset for preventive medicine and secondly, if I recall properly, there have been attempts also towards similar arrangements in the field of HIV infections. It would be worthwhile to find out if those models can be further worked out.

But apart from this, there is probably a new chance for vaccinations against a number of diseases. Vaccination could be a very interesting means for those countries where the health care system is not providing regular medical care at short intervals, which is needed when it comes to sophisticated pharmaceutical treatments.

In addition, since molecular medicine will offer more pharmaceutical treatments for many of those diseases which currently cannot be treated pharmaceutically, there is in principle a possibility to provide large-scale medication to patients in less developed countries if the follow-up of medical treatment is not too demanding with regard to medical infrastructure.

Finally, there is no reason to believe that this molecular medicine – even if prices should be high in the beginning – should not have the same fate as classical treatments already have. After some time on the market there will be a price decay for many of those new compounds as well.

Since the issue is a rather demanding one I would propose that we also think about completely different methods. For example, for those diseases which mainly hit patients in the less developed countries, pharmaceutical industry and non-governmental organizations could come to binding agreements where money is provided for early research and development. This could be an incentive and at the same time reduce the financial risk for the pharmaceutical company. These agreements would mainly apply for early phases of drug discovery and not that much for the later product development, which should be in the responsibility of a pharmaceutical company. The Rockefeller Foundation and Schering have entered into such an agreement recently for the research and early development of male fertility control.

I consider it worthwhile to think along those lines in order to come up with completely new solutions for those demanding problems that we have in certain countries in the world.

4 The Anthropocentric Revolution and Our Common Future

J. Mittelstrass

1 Introduction

A philosopher among scientists – it can be a lonely business, at least as long as philosophy is identified with profundity and science with crude positivism. But things have not looked like that for a long time. Philosophy has accommodated itself to a world which owes ever more to the work of the scientific and technical imagination. And science has learned that reality, even that reality in which scientists work and live, is not confined to what is scientifically the case. Our problems, one might say, do not do us the favour of defining themselves as *either* philosophical *or* scientific. And scientific problems connect with philosophical problems all the more as the world becomes increasingly a product of Man, and as this world begins to appropriate Man to itself, as for instance in biotechnology and reproductive medicine.

Thus the presence of a philosopher at a scientific conference is perhaps something perfectly normal. It is my hope that you will also think so by the end of my lecture. To begin with, I will talk about Man as we have begun to investigate him and to change him from an anthropological perspective, and will then consider what sort of ethics we need to connect scientific progress to a future which is not only human, but also humane.

2 Conditio Humana

Man has always thought of himself both scientifically and philosophically. In the beginning, we have Hippocrates, the physician, and Socrates, the philosopher. In consequence, one can distinguish between a medical or biological anthropology on the one hand, and a philosophical anthropology on the other.

The task and the goal of philosophical anthropology is to determine those *anthropological constants* which, independent of concrete historical and cultural developments, constitute the nature of Man in the sense of providing the constitutive components or properties of being human. The nature (or essence) of Man can be variously conceived, namely, "(1) nature in the sense of biologically (or more generally scientifically) describable dispositions and the behaviour patterns they explain; (2) in the sense of ancient or even prehistoric rules for human action (and possibly also the normative notions that legitimate these rules), and (3) in the sense of Man's 'life world', that is, the experiences available to everyone" (Schwemmer 1980, p 126). What is common to these different approaches to the nature of Man is, in turn, that here (common or similarly applicable) determinations are made which – as *universal* determinations – can be understood as conditions of every historical, cultural and intellectual development of Man, in the form of anthropological constants.

In answer to the objections of *historical* anthropology, which is usually oriented towards the philosophy of history and seeks to represent such constants as properties brought forth by historical developments, let me point out that philosophical anthropology considers properties that even a historical explanation must presuppose as biologically and/or phenomenologically given. Even the appeal to a lifeworld, to historical or to cultural realities has no relativizing consequences. On the contrary, it is precisely the character of the human condition as constituted in the lifeworld that reveals to us on analysis the unavoidable presuppositions of an historical approach. In this sense, a philosophical anthropology embraces historical, cultural, and other empirical aspects – among them the results of physical and historical anthropology, but it attempts either to present their achievements in understanding and explaining as open varieties of a deeper underlying structure of humanity, or to derive them from the analysis of universal presuppositions, i.e. anthropological constants. These in turn are looked for in lifeworld dispositions or, with the same results, elaborated in the form of ethics.

Modern philosophical anthropology takes its point of departure from two opposing conceptions: that due to Max Scheler and that due to Helmut Plessner. According to Scheler, philosophical anthropology is nothing but the quintessence of philosophy itself; according to Plessner it follows the structure of the empirical sciences of Man in the form of an "integrative" discipline. Scheler hearkens back to traditional determinations of Man as *animal rationale;* Plessner is oriented towards the state of biological, medical, psychological, and, in the extended sense, social–scientific research, and he does this with the conceptual goal of a *structural theory* of Man. Common to both in the characterisation of Man is the concept of *world-openness,* which includes the aspect of the openness of human development.

According to Scheler, Man is the "X that can behave in a world-open manner to an unlimited extent" (Scheler 1927, p 49); according to Plessner, Man is characterised by an "eccentric positionality" (Plessner 1928, p 362ff), whereby his eccentric existence, which possesses no fixed centre, is described as the unity of mediated immediacy and natural artificiality. Accordingly, Plessner formulates three *fundamental laws of anthropology* – (1) the Law of Natural Artificiality, (2) the Law of Mediated Immediacy, and (3) the Law of the Utopian Standpoint (Plessner 1928, pp 309–346; see Lorenz 1990, pp 102f). Similarly, Arnold Gehlen states the thesis that Man is by nature a cultural being (Gehlen 1961, p 78), whereby his cultural achievements are seen as compensation for organs and Man is defined as a creature of defect *(Mängelwesen)* (Gehlen 1972, p 37). For Friedrich Nietzsche, Man is the not-yet-determined animal (Nietzsche 1968, p 79), whereby science too is seen as the expression of human endeavour "to determine himself" (Nietzsche 1973, p 533). Furthermore, one of the reasons for the difficulty of saying what Man is lies in the fact that Man is the (only) creature that possesses a reflective relation to itself; that Man, as

Heidegger says, is the creature "which in its being relates understandingly to its being" (Heidegger 1977, pp 52f). This opens up a broad horizon of possible self-interpretations of Man, and to this extent a broad horizon for an answer to the question, What is Man? The only thing that is clear is what can, with regard to the essential openness of Man, be called the *anthropologically basic situation*.

This openness affects all phases of human development, both from an ontogenetic and from a phylogenetic point of view. There is no "natural" fate in the becoming of Man, as an individual or as a species that might be definitely determined by biological laws, even though of course the "schema" of this development is given by certain biological regularities. There is no adulthood before childhood, no reverse ageing, no Achilles who is young until he dies. Only the realisation of these phases is open in the sense explicated, that is to say as a horizon, and not as a predetermined system of paths. In psychological terminology: the architecture of human ontogeny is incomplete (Baltes 1997), and not merely in earlier stages but throughout a lifetime.

It is especially the opposed but complementary concepts, *nature* – or causal relation – and *culture* – or institutional relation – which in this context (in the framework of human ethology) make clear the different but, in the anthropological context, indelibly reciprocal approaches to analysis: "Causal and intentional regularities constitute strictly distinct ranges of objects that must be studied by the disciplines of natural science and cultural science with different scientific methods. Causal regularities are constrained by initial conditions, intentional regularities are determined by goal representations which, due to their social mediation, normally do not become conscious. The disputed question, whether and to what extent sociocultural behaviour is naturally–biologically determined or vice versa is actually a dispute whether some empirically observed behaviour is to be taken as 'natural' (belonging to nature) or as 'cultural' (belonging to culture)" (Lorenz 1990, p 23).

With this it is also clear what kinds of tensions are involved in all forms of philosophical anthropology. These all conceive of themselves rightly (inside and outside philosophy) as fundamental, but also in an integrative sense (similar to Plessner's approach), namely one that takes the knowledge about Man acquired by other (empirical) disciplines into account. Thus even within philosophy, science has its day.

Now it is not my business here to outline our scientific knowledge of Man. This is the province of the sciences themselves, for instance of biology, of psychology and of medicine. But it is important to make clear that the *anthropocentrism* developed within philosophy, according to which Man is the measure of all things, including himself, is a standpoint which has been displaced neither by science nor by philosophy. On the contrary, it is precisely the recent developments in, for instance, biology, which make an anthropocentric standpoint a duty, albeit one which is better expressed in terms of responsibilities (towards nature and oneself) than in terms of domination or control. The place in which anthropology and science meet in this regard – above all anthropology and biology – is the domain of ethics.

3 The Anthropocentric View

Today we are promised great gains above all from the developments of the new biology, for example in medicine and pharmacology, but great risks as well, for instance in the thoughtless or irresponsible application of bioengineering. But this is also not fundamentally new. Discoveries and inventions that point to the future have throughout human history come saddled with dangers and risks of abuse of a new and unimagined order. What may be new in the case of modern biology is the circumstance that developments in biological knowledge appear to place Man in the position of being able to change his own nature, and that this development has consequences for ethics (in the conventional sense). Man intervenes ever more powerfully in evolution, even in his own, and he changes the measures with which he previously described and regulated his situation, that is to say, the human condition (see Mittelstrass 1999).

While we have known since Darwin that Man, not only from the point of view of philosophy and culture but also biologically, has no fixed essence, that – even though this is imperceptible to the individual and only recognisable to science over great periods of time – he is subject to evolutionary changes, indeed that he can intervene in these changes himself, it has only become clear in the light of the new biology that he can deliberately change his own genetic constitution and that of his progeny. In fact, the *conditio humana* itself is changing, in the sense that now even its biological foundations are at Man's disposal. And this creates a completely new and consequential situation for ethics.

There are various consequences that have been drawn for ethics from the results of the new biology. One consequence is the call for a *bioethics,* in the sense of an applied ethics which deals specifically with biological states of affairs. Such a code would prescribe particular watchfulness and particular measures in certain fields, as well as certain applications that could be formulated as rules of an ethics of responsibility. Such rules might include – for instance as applied to developments in genetic technology – both the rule of considering the consequences by carefully checking for possible undesirable results and a rule of caution, which favours the choice of the option that offers the greatest security of prognosis and the least expected harm (see Irrgang 1996, pp 516ff). However, the debate on the ethical problems of biology extends far beyond such bioethics in the direction of *environmental ethics,* which attempts to change the foundations of ethics itself.

The point of departure of such a conception of ethics is often an argument about *going against nature.* According to this, genetic engineering and interventions into human reproductive processes do something that is the business of nature alone; they intervene in a regulatory manner in a self-regulating nature; by gene transfer they cross species boundaries, thus infringing on the "identity of species" (Altner 1991, p 214) and disturb the (relative) stability of ecological balances (Altner 1991, p 217). In arguments of this kind – which also include, by the way, the notion that animals, plants and the elements are like us and we are like them "in the whole of nature" (Meyer-Abich 1984, 24) – we find biological unclarity – what is then the "identity of species"? – coupled with ethical unclarity – what does ethics have to do with the order of species, that is, with biological classifications or even with nature as a whole, however that is to be imagined? Those who think (and write) this way are confusing the empirical (biological states of affairs) with the normative and commit the naturalistic fallacy, that is, they infer what ought to be from what is, they derive norms from facts.

Precisely this is also the case in the well-known arguments of Hans Jonas, who declares the natural to be the highest norm and views any intervention into natural processes as an offence against "naturally" given norms. For example, for Jonas, the technology of cloning is in "contradiction to the dominant strategy of nature" (Jonas 1985, p 179) and thus cannot be justified. The natural – here in the form of a natural reproduction – consequently appears not only as something not to be interfered with (for whatever reasons, for instance, religious reasons) but also as something that pursues its own goals with strategic means and that by these means makes itself the highest normative authority. It is no wonder that this kind of argumentation is often connected with religious themes such as myths of creation. If everything that is natural is creation, the work of a divine creator, then an offence against the natural – in the form of suspending its effects or of making a copy – is an offence against the divine will, which in turn is conceived as norm–giving in a principled sense.

As a matter of fact, the attempt is made repeatedly to construct an ecological ethics on the basis of an inference from facts to norms (which usually reveals a concealed naturalism) and to then oppose this new ethics in the form of *physiocentrism* to the *anthropocentrism* that has long dominated ethics and which is now declared to have been a basic error. A central role in such arguments is played by differing concepts of nature, and thus a bioethics that has been expanded into ecological ethics is also called an ethics of nature. For the anthropocentric position – both in questions of ethics and of nature – Man is the point of departure of all arguments and nature has no intrinsic moral value. For the physiocentric position, nature is characterised by its own (absolute) intrinsic value, which at the same time implies duties of Man toward nature. To be more precise, we can distinguish between *pathocentrism* (all sensible creatures have a moral value), *biocentrism* (all living creatures have a moral value) and *radical physiocentrism* which, as just explained, makes all of nature the bearer of moral value. Common to all these variants is that values, which in fact are always the result of valuations, are declared to be a part of nature itself.

The expansion of a bioethics, a sub-area of applied ethics, to biological ethics in the form of or against the background of physiocentrism is thus based on a misunderstanding. This expansion not only makes ethics dependent on a particular view of the world, but also leads by its naturalistic premises to a new (ethical) *biologism*. Biology is expected to be not only an advisor but also a legislator in ethical affairs. And this in turn involves both a philosophical and a biological misunderstanding, since the new biology teaches us how permeable the boundaries are between the natural and the artificial; that is, those processes determined by Man. The appeal to nature in ethical questions, which made sense in archaic cultures, no longer makes sense here. And one more thing: the notion that moral conduct as a particular form of social behaviour is itself the product of evolution or could be given an evolutionary explanation leads one astray if it is understood in an absolute sense as a foundation of ethics. Whereas in the first case of a biologistic ethics, natural relations are to be taken as the standard of ethics, in the second case ethics would be a product of these relations, and thus our ethical deficits would not be due to the failings of reason but to an evolution that was unfinished and unable to cope adequately with Man (see Wolters 1998; Vogt 1998). An *evolutionary ethics* in this sense would be a convenient excuse for tasks unaccomplished in Man's dealing with himself and with nature.

But these tasks are what have to be addressed – which is why it is only rational ethics, that is, an anthropocentrism in ethics rightly understood, which is able to solve them. Nature gives no ethical lessons, neither in the form of physiocentrism nor in the form of evolutionary ethics. Nature only reminds us when harm is caused; think of environmental problems – of the unfinished tasks of rational ethics.

4 *Homo faber*

In 1488, the Italian philosopher and humanist Giovanni Pico della Mirandola wrote the following about God's intentions towards Man: "We gave you neither a fixed dwelling, Adam, nor a particular appearance, nor any special talent, in order that you might have and own the dwelling, the appearance and the talents that you desire for yourself.... We made you neither heavenly nor earthly, neither mortal nor immortal, so that you might form yourself as your own, worthy, free and creative sculptor" (Pico della Mirandola 1990, pp 5–7). One hundred years later (1596) Johannes Kepler writes in the dedication letter of his *Mysterium cosmographicum:* "We perceive how God, like one of our own architects, approached the task of constructing the universe with order and pattern, and laid out the individual parts accordingly, as if it were not art which imitated nature, but as if God himself had looked to the mode of building of Man who was to be" (Kepler 1981, p 53/55).

What Pico della Mirandola and Kepler still affirm in a pious and expressive language is nothing other than the extension of the concept of Man as *Homo sapiens* to include that of *Homo faber*, both with regard to himself and to his world. The same holds true of the modern epistemological and anthropological developments. Pico della Mirandola's characterisation of Man as "his own sculptor" corresponds to Nietzsche's and the anthropologist Plessner's definition of Man as the not-yet-determined animal, or indeed to Plessner's characterisation of Man by means of his eccentric positionality (which is juxtaposed to the undistanced centricity of the animal). Similarly, Kepler's characterisation of a *Homo faber* competing with God paradigmatically corresponds to the modern notion of scientifically supported technical cultures, in which Man creates and encounters – both in and by means of his productions – not only the world, but indeed himself.

Is Man his own work, in the way that the (modern) world is his work? Certainly not in the sense that Man is an artefact that created itself. For even in his role as *Homo faber*, Man remains bound to his nature, and what is meant by the work-like character of Man is above all his self-determining ("cultural") essence, not his natural essence. Nonetheless, such distinctions, which are also boundaries, are beginning to give. Against the background of modern scientific and technical developments, the possibility has raised its head, that along with the rational nature of Man (that which makes him *Homo sapiens*) we might change not only his external (physical and social) nature but also his internal (biological) nature.

Will Man put at his own disposal all the "parts" that make up his essence – body, soul and reason? Has he become master of his own nature in a sense which would have been unimaginable even for Pico della Mirandola or Kepler? I think that we must accustom ourselves to the fact that this disposal of Man over himself will increase, driven as it is by scientific and technical development. But we must at the same time preserve, in opposition to this development, those indispensable things which are experienced in love and in happiness, in sickness and in death, and in which, despite the threat of the triumph of *Homo faber* over *Homo sapiens*, an essential part of our humanity is contained. Might this be what Pico della Mirandola meant when he had God say to Man that the latter was created neither heavenly nor earthly, neither mortal nor immortal?

5 Conclusion

Casting a concerned glance on the world, Lichtenberg once remarked: "Why should there not be levels of souls reaching up towards God, such that our world was the work of one of them who did not quite know his business, an attempt?" (Lichtenberg 1971, p 410). One cannot very well follow Lichtenberg's line. The responsibility for the state of the world is ours, and not that of a beginner god. But it is true that the modern world is the work of Man, and that he possibly didn't quite know his business. Let us direct our actions, including, indeed above all, our scientific actions in such a way that we aim at a *humane* world, and do not conduct unreflected experiments either on ourselves, or on the world of our creation.

References

Altner G (1991) Naturvergessenheit: Grundlagen einer umfassenden Bioethik. Wissenschaftliche Buchgesellschaft, Darmstadt

Baltes PB (1997) On the incomplete architecture of human ontogeny: selection, optimization, and compensation as foundation of developmental theory. Am Psychol 52:366–380

Gehlen A (1961) Anthropologische Forschung: Zur Selbstbegegnung und Selbstentdeckung des Menschen. Rowohlt, Reinbek

Gehlen A (1972) Der Mensch: Seine Natur und seine Stellung in der Welt [1940]. Akademische Verlagsgesellschaft Athenaion, Wiesbaden

Heidegger M (1977) Sein und Zeit [1927]. Max Niemeyer, Tübingen

Irrgang B (1996) Genethik. In: Nida-Rümelin J (ed) Angewandte Ethik: Die Bereichsethiken und ihre theoretische Fundierung. Ein Handbuch. Kröner, Stuttgart, pp 510–551

Jonas H (1985) Laßt uns einen Menschen klonieren: Von der Eugenik zur Gentechnologie. In: Jonas H, Technik, Medizin und Ethik: Zur Praxis des Prinzips Verantwortung. Insel, Frankfurt

Kepler J (1981) Mysterium Cosmographicum/The Secret of the Universe. Abaris Books, New York

Lichtenberg GC (1971) Schriften und Briefe. Vol II. Carl Hanser, Munich

Lorenz K (1990) Einführung in die philosophische Anthropologie. Wissenschaftliche Buchgesellschaft, Darmstadt

Meyer-Abich KM (1984) Wege zum Frieden mit der Natur: Praktische Naturphilosophie für die Umweltpolitik. Hanser, Munich

Mittelstrass J (1999) The impact of the new biology on ethics. Eur Rev Interdiscipl J Acad Eur 7:277–283

Nietzsche F (1968) Jenseits von Gut und Böse [1886]. In: Colli G, Montinari M (eds) Nietzsche F, Werke: Kritische Gesamtausgabe. Vol VI/2. de Gruyter, Berlin, New York

Nietzsche F (1973) Nachgelassene Fragmente Frühjahr 1881 bis Sommer 1882. In: Colli G, Montinari M (eds) Nietzsche F, Werke: Kritische Gesamtausgabe. Vol V/2. de Gruyter, Berlin, New York

Pico della Mirandola G (1990) De hominis dignitate/Über die Würde des Menschen. Meiner, Hamburg

Plessner H (1928) Die Stufen des Organischen und der Mensch: Einleitung in die philosophische Anthropologie. de Gruyter, Berlin, Leipzig

Scheler M (1927) Die Stellung des Menschen im Kosmos. Otto Reichl, Darmstadt

Schwemmer O (1980) Anthropologie. In: Mittelstrass J (ed) Enzyklopädie Philosophie und Wissenschaftstheorie. Vol I. Bibliographisches Institut, Mannheim, Vienna, Zurich (revised Metzler, Stuttgart, Weimar), pp 126–129

Vogt M (1998) Evolution/Evolutionstheorie(n) 2.3. In: Korff W, et al (eds) Lexikon der Bioethik. Vol I. Gütersloher Verlagshaus, Gütersloh, pp 717–721

Wolters G (1998) Evolution/Evolutionstheorie(n) 2.2. In: Korff W, et al (eds) Lexikon der Bioethik. Vol I. Gütersloher Verlagshaus, Gütersloh, pp 714–717

5 The Contraceptive Technology Revolution

M.F. Fathalla

1 Egon Diczfalusy and the Contraceptive Technology Revolution

Professor Diczfalusy made significant scientific contributions to the development of modern contraceptive technology. But to him, contraceptive technology was not an end in itself. It was a means to an end: better life for *all* people. To him also, contraceptive technology was not to stop with the development of a range of good methods. Research and development had to continue to keep pace with the new frontiers opening up in science. Contraceptive use is a socially responsible reproductive behaviour. People who adopt this responsible reproductive behaviour do not deserve good contraceptives; they deserve the best which science can offer.

In line with what motivated Diczfalusy's work in this field, I will attempt to deal with three aspects of the subject: a brief review of the contraceptive technology revolution from a user's perspective, the impact the technology had on people's lives, and then the needs and the promise for the future.

2 Contraceptive Technology: Past and Present

2.1 Contraception: An Old Human Need

In almost every culture, historians have found ancient, traditional methods that women have used. An Egyptian papyrus dating from 1850 b.c. refers to plugs of honey, gum acacia, and crocodile dung used as a contraceptive vaginal paste (Speroff and Darney 1992). The biblical story of Onan spilling his seed on the ground is probably the most ancient written record of the contraceptive practice of withdrawal (Gen. 38:8–10). For a long time in human history, withdrawal was the only reasonably effective method available, and it was only available to men. Women have had at their disposal only one genuinely effective biological method to postpone pregnancy – prolonged breastfeeding.

2.2 Traditional Contraceptive Approaches

In the more recent past, traditional approaches to contraception gave mainly only one of two choices: to use coitus-related methods (condom and withdrawal for the man; diaphragm, cervical cap, and vaginal spermicides for the woman; periodic abstinence for the couple) with their inconvenience and relative lack of effectiveness, or to use an effective but permanent method (male and female sterilization).

2.3 The Contraceptive Technology Revolution

It was only in the second half of the twentieth century that the approaches to contraception have been dramatically expanded. We had a contraceptive technology revolution. From the point of view of the contraceptive user, this technology revolution offered a number of significant features (Fathalla 1999a). First, contraception was moved outside the bedroom by the development of methods that are not coitus-related and that are used systemically. Second, the development of long-acting methods gave people another choice. They no longer had to make the choice only between methods to be used at every coitus or a permanent method. They could choose a reversible contraceptive method that is effective for one month, two months, three months, five years or ten years. Third, women had access to temporary contraceptive methods that are effective; they no longer needed to use only a permanent method if they wanted to secure effectiveness. In addition, methods of sterilization, male and female, became more simple and safe as out-patient procedures.

But perhaps the most important advantage of the contraceptive technology revolution was that, for the first time in human history, women had at their disposal methods they can use without the need for cooperation of their partners. When they had control of their own fertility, they had control of their lives. A woman, throughout human history, has been subjected to reproductive subordination. She could claim ownership of her head, neck, arms, legs, etc., but a certain part of her body belonged more to certain males of the species, moralists, politicians and lawyers, all of whom decided how this area was best utilized. With the empowerment of the contraceptive technology revolution, a woman can reclaim that part as her own.

3 Contraceptive Technology: The Impact

The impact of the contraceptive technology revolution on people's lives cannot be underestimated. The impact has been overwhelmingly positive. However, some concerns have also been voiced and need to be addressed.

3.1 On the Positive Side

3.1.1 Contraceptive Use

The fruits of the contraceptive technology revolution have been and are being enjoyed by hundreds of millions of people all around the world, people living in the most varied circumstances: in the skyscrapers of

Table 1. World contraceptive use 1998 (United Nations 1999)

	Couples in reproductive ages in 1995[a]	Level of contraceptive use (%)
World	982.2	58
Less developed regions	799.2	55
More developed regions	183.0	70

[a]In millions.

Table 2. Level of current contraceptive use (%) (United Nations 1999)

	World	Less developed regions	More developed regions
Total	58	55	70
Female sterilization	19	21	9
Male sterilization	4	4	5
Pill	8	6	17
IUD	13	14	6
Condom	4	2	14
Other	11	7	21

Manhattan; in peri-urban slums in South America; in rural communities of the Indian subcontinent; people in all socio-economic strata; people with different cultures, religious beliefs and value systems; and people postponing a first pregnancy, spacing children, or putting a limit to childbearing.

Of the 982.2 million couples in reproductive ages in the world in 1995, the level of contraceptive use was estimated at 58% (Table 1). In less developed regions, the level was 55%. In more developed regions, the level was 70%.

The contraceptive method mix varies widely in the world (Table 2). It is interesting, however, to note that in general the overall prevalence of the use of the more modern clinic and supply methods does not differ much between developed and developing regions. The higher contraceptive prevalence in more developed regions is largely accounted for by a relatively more prevalent use of other methods.

3.1.2 Fertility Decline

Parallel to the expansion in contraceptive use, fertility levels continued to decline. Estimations for the year 2000 put the total fertility rate (a measure of the total number of births a woman is expected to have over a lifetime) at 2.9. For more developed regions, the estimate was 1.5. For less developed regions, the estimate was 3.2. If we exclude China, the figure was 3.7 (Population Reference Bureau 2000).

Whatever may have been the factors that prompted the reproductive *evolution* to a small family norm, it was the contraceptive technology *revolution* which helped people to implement their reproductive intentions.

3.1.3 Beyond Demography

The late Jim Grant, Executive Director of UNICEF, made the following statement: "Family planning could bring more benefits to more people at less cost than any other single "technology" now available to the human race. But it is not appreciated widely enough that this would still be true even if there were no such thing as a population problem (Grant 1992).

Contraception should not be looked upon as a temporary measure to ease the world population problem. Contraception will be a permanent feature of the way of life of all succeeding generations on this planet. Our reproductive function is being voluntarily adapted to dramatic new realities. What we are witnessing is a major evolutionary jump that is science-mediated rather than brutally imposed by nature (Fathalla 1997). *Homo sapiens* has escaped the grip of nature in evolution to become a self-evolving animal. The recent dramatic evolution in human reproductive behaviour is not followed or accompanied by a change in the anatomy and/or function of the reproductive system, as would have been expected in other major evolutionary jumps mediated by Mother Nature. As a consequence, *Homo sapiens* has to accomplish its reproductive evolution while retaining a reproductive system geared to high fertility. Women, or their partners, have to use contraception. Women have a span of about 30 reproductive years, during which they were meant by Nature to get pregnant. If women are to bear only one or two children, they will spend only 1–3 years in childbearing. For the remaining years, they, or their partners, will have to lead a contraceptive life if they are to remain sexually active.

3.1.4 The Winners: Women

Fertility by choice, not by chance, is a basic requirement for women's health, well-being and quality of life (Fathalla 1993a). A woman who does not have the means or the power to regulate and control her fertility cannot be considered in a "state of complete physical, mental and social well-being", the definition of health in the constitution of the World Health Organization. She cannot have the joy of a pregnancy that is wanted, avoid the distress of a pregnancy that is unwanted, plan her life, pursue her education, undertake a productive career, or plan her births to take place at optimal times for childbearing, ensuring more safety for herself and better chances for her child's survival and healthy growth and development. With small families now the norm, and with the ability of women to regulate and control their fertility, the woman is finally emerging from behind the mother. Childbearing is becoming *a* function of women, not *the* function of women.

3.2 On the Negative Side

3.2.1 Fertility Control by Women Versus Fertility Control of Women

The contraceptive technology revolution has not been without drawbacks. It lent itself to potential abuse. Contraceptives are meant to be used by women to empower them, to maximize their choices, to give them control on their fertility, and thus their lives. Contraceptives, particularly long-acting and the now simplified permanent methods, can be used and have been used by governments and others to control rather than empower women. Some governments were short-sighted not to see that when women are given a real choice, and the information and means to implement their choices, they will make the most rational decisions for themselves, for their communities and ultimately for the world at large.

It must be pointed out that as far as health and human rights are concerned, there is little to choose between coerced contraception, sterilization or abortion, because society does not want the child, and coerced motherhood, because society wants the child.

In 1976, the national population policy of India permitted state legislatures to enact laws for compulsory sterilization. During the following national emergency period, it was reported that several million forced sterilizations were performed (Andorka 1990).

The opposite side of the same coin is the declaration of Nicolae Ceausescu that "the foetus is the socialist property of the whole society. Giving birth is a patriotic duty.... Those who refuse to have children are deserters, escaping the law of natural continuity" (Hord et al. 1991).

Romania under Ceausescu may have been an extreme example of coerced motherhood. But coerced motherhood or compulsory child-bearing, broadly defined, is a major problem in the world today. Women are coerced into childbearing when they are denied the choice, when they are denied the means to avoid unwanted pregnancy, and when society makes children the only goods a woman can deliver and is expected to deliver. In many societies in the world today, women are left with no choice in life except to pursue a reproductive career.

3.2.2 *Contraceptive Technology and the Pandemic of Sexually Transmitted Infections*

It has been sometimes claimed that the availability of modern contraceptive technology has encouraged a sexual behaviour that led to the pandemic of sexually transmitted infections, or at least it has decreased the reliance on the condom as a method of contraception that also protects against infection. This was an argument often made in Japan, to delay the introduction of oral contraceptives. There is no scientific data to support this claim. It may be recalled that the continent most hit by the sexually transmitted infections, including HIV, Africa, is the continent with the lowest contraceptive prevalence.

3.2.3 *Safety Concerns*

As with any drug, an increase in effectiveness is often accompanied by a decrease in the margin of safety. From a public health point of view, contraceptive drugs and devices have an excellent record of safety. They have been used by hundreds of millions of women over extended periods of time and under the most varied circumstances. Few drugs have been, and continue to be, subjected to such rigorous scrutiny with respect to safety. This scrutiny is particularly important because, unlike individuals who use drugs to cure illness, women (and men) who use contraception are taking preventive action (Fathalla 1991).

Safety concerns loom particularly large if a service system is concerned about demographic targets than about the health and welfare of clients. A contraceptive can be safe or unsafe, depending on who is using it and the quality of the service system delivering it. Moreover, the concept of safety must reflect client concerns. Safety cannot be defined simply as the absence of life-threatening complications, but must be assessed from a woman's perspective. So-called minor inconveniences or side-effects may mean a lot to some women who experience them.

3.2.4 Women as Means and Not Ends

A dialogue between users and creators of the technology has been, until recently, lacking. In particular, women were sometimes viewed as means to achieve demographic targets and not ends. The voices of women should not only be heard, but also heeded. Women's health advocates and potential users should be represented in all decision-making mechanisms and advisory bodies that are established to guide the research process.

4 Contraceptive Technology: The Unfinished Agenda

In spite of the major achievements and great impact of the contraceptive technology revolution, we are still left with an unfinished agenda (Fathalla 1993b). The contraceptive technology revolution was made possible through the convergence of three factors. First, there was the sense of need and the clarity of mission, dictated by global demographic concerns. Second, science was ripe with new advances in reproductive biology, and particularly endocrinology. Third, industry, seeing the potential of rapidly expanding markets and the opportunities provided by science, positioned itself for an active role. The stalling of the revolution can be traced to the same three factors. The mission lost its clarity, science began to dry up, and industry, with few exceptions, has retrenched. Product liability, drug regulatory requirements, political climate, perceptions that the market in rich countries is already mature and that the expanding market in developing countries is not rewarding, together with opportunities for drug development in other fields of medicine, all served to put industry off from the field of contraceptive research and development. Few have kept their commitment to this important area of women's health. They deserve credit for it. They will prove to be right in continuing their investment.

The range of contraceptive choices, much broadened by the contraceptive technology revolution, is still inadequate to meet the present and rapidly expanding needs. It is true that improved software, i.e. better healthcare delivery systems, will take us a long way to address this inadequacy, but we still need more hardware. Let us look at the verdict.

4.1 The Unmet Need

As stated in the *Programme of Action of the International Conference on Population and Development*, Cairo, 1994, "…the full range of modern family planning methods still remains unavailable to at least 350 million couples worldwide, many of whom say they want to space or prevent another pregnancy" (United Nations 1994). The available methods of family planning dictate their own delivery systems, and they vary in acceptability and continuation.

4.2 Unwanted Pregnancy and Abortion

Another verdict is given by estimated 46 million women who resort to induced abortion each year – 26 million in countries with liberal abortion laws and 20 million where abortion is restricted or prohibited by law, many of them risking their lives and health in the process (Henshaw et al. 1999). Given the state of the art, contraceptive use cannot prevent all of these abortions. A large number of unwanted pregnancies worldwide result from contraceptive failure.

5 Women Need a Second Contraceptive Technology Revolution

Women have more at stake in fertility control than anyone else. Women struggled and paid a heavy price to claim their right to control their fertility.

Apart from the general need to expand contraceptive choices by more user-controlled and more safe methods, three specific unmet needs are articulated by women's groups (Fathalla 1999b):

- Expanded male contraceptive choices, participation and responsibility
- Woman-controlled methods that provide additional protection against sexually transmitted infections
- Methods which women can use, as a back-up, when exposed to unprotected sexual intercourse, and which will decrease the resort to abortion

5.1 Expanding Male Contraceptive Choices and Responsibility

There is a need for more participation by men in fertility regulation. Women for biological reasons have to carry all the burden and risks of pregnancy and childbirth. This, however, is no reason that they should also carry most of the burden of fertility regulation. Currently worldwide, the burden of contraception is unequally shared, with three times more women than men using contraception (United Nations 1999). Moreover, it is the methods which women use which can be associated with potential side effects. The male has not benefited that much from the contraceptive technology revolution. There is, however, a remarkable gap between the need and demand for novel male contraceptives on the one hand, and the state of development or even the state of basic knowledge about the function of the male contraceptive system on the other. Advances in cell and molecular biology and biotechnology are now providing new tools for studying male reproductive physiology, and identifying potential novel targets for fertility control. A sustained research effort is, however, needed if men are to have broader contraceptive choices to enable them to share effectively in the responsibility for fertility regulation.

5.2 Protection Against Sexually Transmitted Infections

The need for a method which a woman can use to protect herself against sexually transmitted infections, including HIV, has become urgent. The World Health Organization estimated the number of new cases of curable sexually transmitted infections (excluding HIV) in 1995 to be more than 365 millions (World Health Organization 1997). According to a World Bank study quantifying the burden of disease, sexually transmitted diseases (STDs) rank as the second major cause of the disease burden in young adult women in developing countries, accounting for 8.9% of the total disease burden in that age group (World Bank 1993). Among males of the same age group, STDs are not among the top ten causes and account only for 1.5% of the disease burden. For a mix of biological and social reasons, women are more likely to be infected, are less likely to seek care, are more difficult to diagnose, are at more risk for severe disease sequelae, and are more subject to social discrimination and consequences. This is in addition to the risk of transmitting infection to the foetus from an infected mother. The most effective method available for protection against STDs, the condom, is controlled by men. Available female barrier methods either lack in effectiveness or acceptability. Another problem which women face is that there is no method which can protect from infection but would allow them to get pregnant. It is quite common, at least in developing countries, for women to get the infection from their husbands who have multiple sexual partners. The need is for an effective method, a vaginal microbicide, which women can use and control without the necessity for partner cooperation. It is possible that if such a method becomes available, women will do better than men in compliance, providing more hope for the control of the pandemic of sexually transmitted infections.

5.3 "Retroactive Contraception"

The global drama of unsafe abortion has reached a dimension that can no longer be neglected. The World Health Organization estimates that millions of women around the world risk their lives and health to end an unwanted pregnancy. Every day, 55,000 unsafe abortions take place –

95% of them in developing countries – and lead to the death of more than 200 women daily (World Health Organization 1998).

The Program of Action adopted by the Cairo International Conference on Population and Development in 1994 (United Nations 1994) stressed that "every attempt should be made to eliminate the need for abortion". Partly because of the realities of present gender power relationships, women are often exposed to unprotected sexual intercourse. Women need backup methods which they can use in such instances to decrease the need for induced abortion. These include emergency contraception (to be used within 72–120 h of intercourse), luteal contraception (to be used in the second half of the menstrual cycle) and menses-inducers to be used at the expected time of menstruation. This "retroactive contraception" would also be suited to the particular needs of adolescents where the decision to contracept is often made post-coitally. It will also be needed in refugee situations. The advent of anti-progestins and a better understanding of the process of implantation of the fertilized ovum have improved the prospects for the development of retroactive contraception.

6 The Promise for the Future

Will women get the contraceptives they still need to pursue their reproductive rights and reproductive health? Science is ripe for a contraception-21 initiative. Advances in cell and molecular biology have opened new frontiers that have yet to be exploited for the development of new contraceptive approaches (Harrison and Rosenfield 1996). But only industrial resources can make it happen. I applaud Schering AG as one of the few major international pharmaceutical companies that give priority to women's health, and who can make it happen.

References

Andorka R (1990) The use of direct incentives and disincentives and of indirect social economic measures in fertility policy and human rights. In: Population and Human Rights. United Nations, New York, p 132

Fathalla MF (1991) Contraceptive technology and safety. Popul Sci 10:7–26

Fathalla MF (1993a) Contraception and women's health. Br Med Bull 49:245–251

Fathalla MF (1993b) The unfinished revolution. Populi Oct:8–10

Fathalla MF (1997) Global trends in women's health. Int J Gynecol Obstet 58:5–12

Fathalla MF (1999a) Contraception-21. Int J Gynecol Obstet 67 [Suppl 2]:5–13

Fathalla MF (1999b) Contraception and the unmet needs of women. Gynaecol Forum 4:25–27

Henshaw SK, Singh S, Haas T (1999) The incidence of abortion worldwide. Int Fam Plann Perspect 25:S30–S38

Grant JP (1992) The state of the world's children 1992. UNICEF. Oxford University Press, New York, p 58

Harrison PF, Rosenfield A (1996) Contraceptive research and development: looking to the future. National Academy, Washington D.C., pp 2,9

Hord C, David HP, Donnay F, Wolf M (1991) Reproductive health in Romania: reversing the Ceausescu legacy. Stud Fam Plann 22:231

Population Reference Bureau (2000). 2000 World Population Data Sheet. Population Reference Bureau, Washington D.C.

Speroff L, Darney PD (1992) A Clinical guide for contraception. Williams and Wilkins, Baltimore, p 184

United Nations (1994) Report of the International Conference on Population and Development (Cairo, 5–13 September 1994). United Nations A/Conf.171/13, New York, pp 7.13, 8.25

United Nations (1999) World Contraceptive Use 1998 Data sheet. United Nations. Department of Economic and Social Affairs. Population Division. New York. UN Publication (ST/ESA/SER.A/175) Sales No. E.99.XIII.4-ISBN 92-1-151330-8

World Bank (1993) World Development Report 1993 – investing in health. Oxford University Press, New York, p 215

World Health Organization (1997) The world health report 1997. World Health Organization, Geneva, p 15

World Health Organization (1998) World health day 1998 fact sheets – prevent unwanted pregnancy. WHD 98.9. World Health Organization, Geneva, p 1

Round Table Discussions

6 Novel Insight into Hormonal Control of Reproduction and Ageing

Chair: R. Ivell
Participants: A.O. Brinkmann, A.C.B. Cato, J. Herbert, H. Hoshiai, O.A. Jänne, L. Martini, F. Naftolin, C. Rivier, G. Telegdy

1 Introduction

R. Ivell

We are celebrating Prof. Egon Diczfalusy's 80th birthday. In his lifetime he has seen a dramatic change in the way we think about disease and how to control it. One needs to consider the knowledge of our field in the first half of the twentieth century to appreciate this: it was a world devoid of antibiotics and pure pharmaceutical compounds, a world which did not have immunoassays, and certainly knew virtually nothing about DNA and everything we now understand by the terms molecular biology or biotechnology. What we should, therefore, consider in this discussion are not just ideas which could become realistic in the next 5 years or so, but also visions of a future world with changes and revolutions as dramatic as Professor Diczfalusy has seen in his lifetime. We should also think about whether we want the changes that are possible. In this way scientists need the "utopian standpoint" referred to by Prof. Mittelstrass, with a vision of the future, but also with a notion of how to get there in small steps. Partly, as Prof. Benagiano pointed out, much of what we need to do is simply to spread what we already know to the rest of the world, to apply the skills and information we already have. But we are still presented with many knowledge barriers which need first to be surpassed.

One possible vision is of a holistic approach to understanding and manipulating the body. Television has provided us with a Star-Trek hero in Dr. Pilla McCoy, who is seen to use a scanner – his "tricorder" – which offers instant holistic appraisal of bodily functions, is comprehensive and yet non-invasive. Is this still mythology, or could we be getting close to such an approach. The Human Genome Project will soon provide us with a list of all the human genes, and hopefully also their mode and pattern of expression (functional genomics). We shall also soon be able to consider the majority of proteins made in different tissues (proteomics), though this will take a little longer. I like to think that in the not too distant future we shall have technologies available (microchips) which will allow us to use this knowledge to gather a fingerprint of human physiology, comparing one organ with another, comparing health with disease, and to do this in a holistic fashion, using bioinformatics, where the whole pattern of expression registered by such chips has more information than the sum of the individual reactions. In this way we should have a technique available, albeit not yet non-invasive, which would give us the molecular equivalent of the histological section, which to the experienced eye of the pathologist contains a complete picture of health and disease though devoid of molecular labels. Here major questions for the future are whether this technology can be made cheaply and for routine application? Can it become more or less non-invasive? And what role does individual variation play in all this? Will we be able to get a view of the forest in spite of all the individual trees?

In reproductive medicine the early embryo has at last become accessible, and in certain countries it is possible to begin looking at early regulatory events. Will it be possible to manipulate the embryo by activation or silencing of embryonic genes, in this way offering ways of later influencing fertility or prolonging health expectancy? This is clearly a topic fraught with ethical implications, but nonetheless worth discussing, as is any notion of manipulating the human germ-line or somatic cells from early development onwards. Given the continued – though not irrevocable – setbacks in gene therapy approaches, how realistic is such a very fine-tuned manipulation of cells in the body for healthy individuals? And, of course, do we need it?

Pharmacology has been preoccupied in the last decades with the vision of the "magic bullet." These are single pure compounds which can achieve an unambiguous alteration in physiology or a disease state. Given the ideas of endocrine networks and informational redundancy that we now have, it is clear that such approaches are limited. We need now to think about pharmacological specificity as the resultant of several less specific events. Modern ideas about the transcriptional regulation of genes shows that it might be possible to get very specific effects in cells by addressing different combinations of transcription factors and their cofactors. We need first to understand the codes by which a specific cell switches on a specific gene, using combinations of molecules which individually have only limited specificity. At the larger level, we might be able to take the holistic approach one step further, and by influencing a molecule or cell in one part of the body, achieve a specific effect in a quite different organ, using the body's own endocrine networks to integrate and process the biological information. In this way, it might be possible to provide a scientific basis for many of the currently frowned upon natural or alternative therapies, and for psychosomatic effects, and develop these further.

In this future world, modern techniques of genomics and bioinformatics will play a central role, but if we are clever, then these should in turn lead on to simpler, less invasive therapies. And in the same way that discrete drug application has done away with primitive surgery, we should be able to expect that simple and non-invasive manipulations in the far future (e.g., mixtures of substances, acupuncture, psychotherapy, etc.) might be able to replace very high-tech and expensive procedures in the present and near future.

In this Round Table Discussion, the participants have been asked to comment on some of the following questions: How do we see the role of modern genomics and proteomics influencing the way we diagnose and treat people, or consider supplementation treatments? Given all the new information that we have from the Human Genome Project, will this open up possibilities for more indirect forms of treatment, for example, influencing the stress axis to regulate fertility? Related to this topic, what opportunities do you think we shall have to influence mental problems in new ways, particularly in aging, but also in other circumstances? Modern bioscience is also providing detailed structural information on pharmacological target molecules. How can this be used to design newer types of reagents?

2 Role of Modern Genomics and Proteomics: Part I

A.O. Brinkman

2.1 Development of a New Kind of Hormone

With respect to modulation of hormone action, I expect exciting new developments in protein 3D structure information, particularly hormone receptor structures (for steroids, gonadotrophins, growth hormone and growth factors). This 3D structure information will not only reveal insight into the active and inactive receptor forms, but also provide knowledge on interacting surfaces available for interacting partners, co-activators, co-repressors, and tissue-specific receptor modulators. In addition and most important in this respect is that information on the 3D interaction surfaces induced by the hormone/antihormone will predict the complementary interacting surface structures of possible known and unknown new protein partners. In this way it will be feasible to design in the future completely new types of hormones and antihormones (="receptor-activating/-inactivating ligands") which shape the correct/incorrect 3D structure of the receptor not by interacting with the classical ligand-binding pocket or domain, but at other interacting surfaces. A first attempt has been successfully applied for the estrogen receptor by the use of small peptides.

2.2 Unraveling Tissue-Specific Action of Hormones

The use in the near future of human embryonic stem cell lines will reveal information on factors and processes involved in tissue differentiation and their modulation. The next step will be the development of all kinds of different hormone target cell lines, including those of different parts of the reproductive tract, of the hypothalamus and pituitary, but also an important number of yet unrecognized target cell lines from all kinds of different tissues. These cell lines are excellent tools for the testing and development of new drugs, hormones, receptor modulators for their normal tissue-specific action (agonists) or abnormal tissue-specific action ("side effects" and/or antagonists) as well as modulating environmental factors for their interference in normal processes.

2.3 Identification of Hormone Receptor Variants in Health and Disease

After completion of the Human Genome Project and the identification of all the functional implications of the different genes (including those of the known hormone receptors as well as new hormone receptors) information will be become available on all kind of variants acting in a normal situation and in pathological situations. The structural information on receptor proteins will provide complete elucidation of their role in hormone action. Aberrant structures will be created and tested for their functionality and linkage to a phenotype in conditional knock-out systems. In this way, a molecular basis will be created for so-called idiopathic hormonal diseases. Already several examples are currently known for steroid receptors (androgen, mineralocorticoid).

3 Role of Modern Genomics and Proteomics: Part II

A.C.B. Cato

3.1 Sexual Differentiation and Other Post-natal Physiological Processes

Modern genomics and proteomics have now put us in the field of "hypothesis-free" search for genes regulated by different hormonal and environmental cues. We are going to isolate genes in different signal transduction pathways that we never thought were related in any way. This will open up for us several possibilities for interfering with distinct pathways for therapeutic purposes. We will also be in a position to specifically investigate changes in the expression of genes and proteins involved in defined physiological and pathophysiological situations.

In this connection I would like to draw attention to one of the unanswered questions that have been posed for many years in the field of androgen action in sexual differentiation and in the regulation of several physiological processes during postnatal life. From the existence of two androgens (testosterone and dihydrotestosterone), it has been argued that two receptors rather than just one receptor exist for androgen action. While current molecular biological experiments point to the existence of only one androgen receptor, other studies show otherwise. The pharmacological survey of binding of dihydrotestosterone in several tissues of the beagle dog and studies on androgen-dependent developmental transformations in the larynx of male *Xenopus laevis* are some of the many examples that suggest the existence of more than one androgen receptor. Other evidence includes the binding of both 5α- and 5β-dihydrotestosterone to avian and mouse osteoblasts. These controversies have so far not been resolved. We now hope that with the recent developments in the field of genomics and proteomics we will get clearer answers as to whether more than one androgen receptor exists to explain the various observations made on androgen action.

When it became clear from previous experiments that steroid receptors regulated gene expression, it was thought that just the receptors and DNA were enough for this purpose. We now know that receptor-associating proteins known as co-activators and co-repressors are needed for the modulation of the action of steroid receptors. So far, not all these modulating proteins have been identified and there are still questions on the specificity of their interaction in defined tissues. These questions will be answered, we hope, with the recent developments in proteomics. The next task will then be to identify the biological function of the co-activators and co-repressors. This can be achieved by targeted disruption of the genes that code for these proteins. In future, we are not only going to see the technique of gene knock-out being very popular but we are going to experience targeted disruption of genes in distinct cells and at predefined stages. This will help us tremendously in finding out the functions of proteins in the environment in which they are expressed and will contribute to the search of novel compounds to interfere with their action.

3.2 Modern Bioscience and New Types of Reagents

When we look at steroid receptors, the X-ray structural studies that have been carried out in the past have provided useful starting points in the determination of molecules that will or will not bind to the receptors. However, there are improvements needed for clearer decisions to be made as to which ligands will be agonists or antagonists. When we talk of glucocorticoids, for example, we need to know which ligands that bind to the receptor exhibit dissociating activities that will distinguish transactivation from transrepression. As the crystal structural analyses carried out so far have been made with portions of receptors lacking interacting factors, it will be important to devise newer techniques for a more complete view of the receptors. This will allow us to see the receptors with their interacting co-activators or co-repressors and thereby provide a complete picture of the receptors in their folded configuration. Unfortunately, current structural studies are only feasible with individual molecules or pairs of molecules or at most a group of three. Anything more than this becomes impossible to crystallize. The challenge for the future is, therefore, to find means of obtaining detailed structures of steroid receptors with associating proteins.

Steroid receptors such as the glucocorticoid, mineralocorticoid, or androgen receptors reside in the cytoplasm in their non-activated states and become transported into the nucleus upon ligand binding. This translocation process can be disrupted with molecules that affect the movement of the receptors without necessarily interacting with their ligand-binding domains. This will open an area of interference of action of steroid receptors in a non-classical manner via the use of inhibitors of cytoplasmic–nuclear transport. Such an approach can only be feasible if we have sufficient information on the factors that interact with the receptors and that influence their transport in and out of the nucleus. Various techniques such as tagging the receptors with fluorescence proteins combined with real-time imaging analysis and photobleaching studies (FLIP and FRAP) will be necessary for determining the intracellular movement of the receptors. Such information will be needed for designing a way of controlling the cytoplasmic–nuclear transport of the receptors.

4 New Opportunities to Influence Mental Problems

L. Martini

4.1 Role of Progestational Agents in the Elderly

It is known that the conductance of peripheral nerves deteriorates with aging and that this is accompanied by a considerable degradation of the protecting myelin sheath. We have recently shown that the major biochemical changes occurring with aging in the myelin of peripheral nerves (e.g. the sciatic nerve of the rat) are due to the drop of two crucial proteins, specific of the peripheral myelin: namely protein Po and protein PMP22.

We have now shown that pretreatment of aging rats with progesterone (P) and dihydroprogesterone (DHP) prevents the age-related loss of these proteins. Consequently, we have suggested that this effect may be linked to the classical mechanism of action of progesterone, since the sciatic nerve possesses progesterone receptors (PR). The peripheral myelin originates from the Schwann cells, which represent the glial elements of the peripheral nervous system (PNS). We have then prepared pure cultures of rat Schwann cells and measured the production of proteins Po and PMP22 in the presence or absence of P, DHP, and tetrahydroprogesterone (THP). It appeared that progestational agents may increase the production of these proteins acting directly in Schwann cells which, incidentally, express the PR. These studies underline a possible role of progestational agents in protecting the PNS from the deteriorating events of aging.

5 Non-reproductive Action of Reproductive Hormone: Possible Therapeutical Application

G. Telegdy

It has been shown that a number of reproductive peptide hormones elicit action which has nothing to do with their original actions. For example, superactive analogue of luteinizing hormone-releasing hormone (LH-

RH) has antitumor action and it can be used for treating prostatic cancer, etc. LH-RH has also amnesic action, meaning it impairs learning and memory functions.

In the last few years at our department, we have concentrated on the action of another reproductive hormone, namely oxytocin, on certain behavior, for example on learning and memory function. We have demonstrated that oxytocin has amnesic action in experimental animals – in rats – impairing learning and memory function. Following this line, we supposed that if elicit drugs acting on this level is a certain type of learning phenomenon, than the action should be influenced by oxytocin. Indeed, oxytocin could attenuate the development of acute tolerance of morphine, heroin, enkephalin and beta-endorphin. Oxytocin attenuated the chronic tolerance to morphine and decreased the heroin self-administration. This action is mediated by dopamine receptors because the dopamine receptor antagonist, pimozide, could prevent the action of oxytocin. A number of C-terminal fragments of oxytocin, even the dipeptide of the C-terminal, which does not carry the action of oxytocin, still can have beneficial action on acute tolerance.

At present, the major problem in the treatment of drug dependency is the handling of withdrawal signs. We have tested, also in rats, the influence oxytocin or some fragments of oxytocin has on precipitated withdrawal syndrome. Central and peripheral administration of oxytocin attenuated the withdrawal sign and fragments and analogues such as Z-PGlu-L-Leu and Z-Gln-L-leu were the most active compounds attenuating the withdrawal signs. Oxytocin decreases the cocaine-induced stereotype reaction also.

These data indicate that oxytocin might act on drug addictive reactions, and compounds which derive from oxytocin might be considered to have therapeutical action in addictive reactions in patients as well.

6 Closing Remarks

R. Ivell

We are at the beginning of a new century, and a new era of medical treatment, especially thanks to the Human Genome Project. This will also be an era of rapidly changing demography. Will we be able to grow old but stay healthy? And will we shift the priority of human existence from one of keeping healthy and disease-free to one of how can we afford it and who can afford it? One thing that is clear is that we are still very ignorant and that much of what we read in current textbooks will need to be rewritten. But this means that there will be new fields for research and application, and most importantly we shall not only be opening new doors, but probably discovering whole new buildings.

7 Contraception: New Approaches and Future Perspectives

Chair: D.T. Baird
Participants: B. Affandi, D.F. Archer, G. Bialy, W. Boonkasemsanti, P.G. Crosignani, H.B. Croxatto, H.L. Gabelnick, L. Kovács, W. Oelkers

1 Introduction

D.T. Baird

1.1 Contraception at the End of the Twentieth Century

In the last 30 years there has been a striking increase in the prevalence of the use of contraception worldwide which has had a significant impact in slowing the rate of increase in population growth. During this time there has been no totally new form of contraception since the introduction of the pill in the early 1960s. However, new delivery systems for hormonal contraception have allowed some progress to be made in the development of long-acting methods such as implants. The introduction of new progestogens such as drospirenone holds some promise for reducing side-effects which interfere with acceptability and continuation rates. There is an interesting variation in the use and acceptability of the available hormonal methods in different parts of the world. While the combined oral contraceptive pill is very popular in Western Europe, it is little used in China and hardly at all in Japan. Injectables are very popular in South Africa while implants are becoming widely used in Indonesia. These differences are probably due to a combination of preference of providers, users and users' partners. Since the 1990s there has been a resurrection in the popularity of condoms largely due to the wish to protect against STDs including AIDS. For the same reason there is now a massive research investment in microbicides.

Even with a wide choice of freely available contraceptive methods, it is inevitable that there will still be a need for access to safe abortion. The introduction of medical abortion offers the potential to provide choice and a wide availability of safe abortion in both developing and developed countries. If contraceptive failure is recognised soon enough, emergency contraception may prevent unwanted pregnancy. However it will only have a significant impact on the incidence of unplanned pregnancy if it is readily available and "no longer the world's best kept secret".

1.2 Contraception in the Twenty-first Century

It is likely that new contraceptive methods in the twenty-first century will not only be highly effective but confer additional health benefits such as the reduction in blood loss associated with the levonorgestrel-releasing intrauterine system (IUS).

To a reproductive biologist the most challenging prospect is the possibility of interfering non-selectively with reproductive processes. Selective receptor modulators of progesterone (PRMs) oestrogen (SERMs) and possibly androgens are likely to be developed in the next 10 years for the treatment of disease of the reproductive system and as hormone replacement in both men and women. It is likely that their use as contraceptives will have additional health benefits. For example, the substitution of SERMs for ethinyl oestradiol should reduce the small risk of breast cancer associated with the use of the combined oral contraceptive pill.

Another theoretically attractive approach to selective interference with reproductive processes is immunocontraception. There is a wide range of potential targets including those involved in interaction between the sperm and the egg and embryo and the uterus. For example, we have known for over 30 years that immunisation against human chorionic gonadotropin (hCG) produces sterility in experimental monkeys. However, fear of the possibility of provoking autoimmune consequences as a result of immunisation against natural substances and the political fear about potential misuse has inhibited research in this area. For these reasons there is little commercial activity or enthusiasm for immunocontraceptives.

Last but not least it is likely that with the first decade of the twenty-first century we will see the marketing of hormonal contraception for men. Research in this area has been hampered by the perceived lack of acceptability of such a method to men and to their partners. However, the recent surveys demonstrating in a number of cultures that men would welcome such a method probably reflects the increasing acceptance of the male in matters of reproductive health. In addition, an emerging interest and enthusiasm for hormone replacement therapy for men has accelerated the development of better preparations of androgens which are essential for new male contraceptives.

The same symbiosis has stimulated the development of partnerships between private commercial companies and public sector organisations.

2 Injectable Contraception

B. Affandi

Available data indicate that the most important problem with currently available contraceptive methods is the unmet need (Table 1) of "reproductive-age couples who do not plan to have a pregnancy yet they do not use any contraceptive method at all". The reasons for people not using contraceptive methods may be divided into two main categories: the problem of logistics and the problem of performance. Experience has shown that every new contraceptive method attracts a new group of acceptors who would probably not otherwise have used a contraceptive method at all. The above facts strongly suggest that there is indeed a major need for the development of a variety of contraceptive methods to suit the different requirements of the different starts of society.

Injectable contraception is very popular in developing countries like Indonesia (Table 2). In order to improve the acceptability of injectable contraception, we must address its disadvantages, i.e. menstrual disturbances and dependency on health provider, and enhance the advantages (Table 3).

Table 1. Unmet need – reproductive-age couples who do not want pregnancy yet do not use any contraceptive method

Reproductive-age couples
- Do not want pregnancy
- Yet do not use any contraceptive method

Range
- 6%–45%

Caused by
- Logistic problems
- The method

Fathalla: "…every new contraceptive method attracts certain new users who otherwise will not use any contraceptive method at all"

Table 2. Contraceptive mix, Indonesia, March 2000

Methods	*n*	%
Injectables	9,743,550	35.2
Pills	7,796,474	28.1
IUDS	5,218,196	18.8
Implants	3,156,705	11.4
Sterilisation	1,515,406	5.5
Others	278,473	1.0
Total	27,708,804	100.0

Table 3. Injectable contraception

Advantages	Disadvantages
Long-acting	Menstrual disturbance
Highly effective	Given by health provider
Safe	
Noncontraceptive benefits	
Reversible	
"Potent medicine"	
Contact health provider	
No oestrogen	

3 Current Evaluation of Immunocontraception

D.F. Archer

3.1 Challenges

The important aspect of immunocontraception relates to the fact that gametes, such as sperm cells and oocytes, have different cellular components compared to somatic cells. They have unique antigenic sites sufficiently different from somatic cells that they could be targeted with a vaccine to produce antibodies or blocking agents that inhibit or reduce fecundity or fertilisability. To this end, immunocontraception and vaccine development is different from that of a vaccine produced to protect the individual from a disease [1]. One of the problems of immunocontraception is that the immune response to self-antigens is difficult to initiate. A second problem is to identify a unique antigenic site on one of the gametes that is entirely different from that found in the other cells of the body. Third, the contraceptive vaccine requires a degree of reversibility. In this regard, the interval between injections of the antigen must be such that there should be a loss of antibody activity that would allow an individual or a couple to have a degree of confidence that their fecundity would not be significantly impaired forever [1].

Contraceptive vaccine development has been fraught with the problem of autoimmunity, particularly related to zona pellucida epitopes [2, 3]. Attempts to develop a specific zona pellucida antibody have resulted in a significant reduction of primary oocytes in animal models, and in rodents there has been associated an acute oophoritis [4–7].

There is also a need for better adjuvants to improve the immunocontraceptive antibody response [8–10].

3.2 Recent Developments

There has been an enhanced interest in immunocontraception because of the recent new knowledge and development in vaccines technology and immunology [1]. Cytokines have been identified that are involved in the regulation of the immune response [9]. The receptor on the T cell for antigenic loci has been identified and will help clarify in the future the function of this receptor in the antigen-antibody response [6, 11]. This information will be useful in the development of an immunocontraceptive vaccine.

Coincident with this information has been the identification of how genes regulate the immune system. Although this information is only beginning to be applicable in the clinical arena, it is an important milestone by identifying genes that could be altered for reducing or augmenting the immune responses to contraceptive vaccines.

The use of molecular biology has increased our ability to synthesise antigens and specific gamete epitopes with properties that could be useful in vaccine development [1, 12, 13].

The ability to insert specific genomic sequences into appropriate vectors may result in the production of large quantities of an antigen that would be available for vaccine development [14].

All of the above innovations translate into an enhanced understanding of the immune and reproductive systems that would be helpful in the development of an immune approach to contraception [1].

3.3 Immunocontraceptive Targets

There are a variety of targets in the reproductive process that have been investigated for immunocontraception. The most common are sperm cell membrane and oocyte zona pellucida proteins [15, 16]. There are a variety of sites on the sperm head that have been identified and targeted for vaccine development [17–23].

Sperm membrane proteins that interact with the zona pellucida are significant targets for immunocontraception. The ability to block the fusion of the sperm membrane with the zona pellucida can be a significant issue for reducing fertilisability [23]. Zona pellucida glycoproteins, known as ZP1, ZP-2 and ZP3, have been identified and have been isolated and studied for their ability to elicit an immune response. ZP3 only becomes apparent in the late stages of follicular development, and is a unique glycoprotein that could be exploited as a potential target for immunocontraception [3, 4, 7, 24–28].

Testes-specific lactic dehydrogenase (LDH)-C4 has been investigated for over 20 years as a potential target for reducing spermatogenesis and altering fertility. Research continues on testes-specific LDH-C4 in primate species [19].

Gonadotropins themselves, human follicle-stimulating hormone (hFSH), luteinising hormone (hLH) and hCG, have individually been utilised for immunocontraception [29, 30]. Attempts to develop an antibody to hFSH and hLH have resulted in limited success. The ability to develop an antibody which is particularly directed to hFSH has been fraught with difficulty. There appears to be a blocking antibody with resultant recovery of hFSH biologic function [22, 31–35].

Of all the protein hormones studies, hCG and its alpha or beta subunits is the most promising lead [30, 36, 37]. HCG is a hormone that is uniquely present only during pregnancy, except in few instances when it has been associated with neoplastic changes in the lung, gastrointestinal tract, and testis [31]. Studies have shown that a vaccine to hCG can be effective. An hCG vaccine has been testing in limited clinical trials [37, 38]. The drawbacks are the inability to mount a persistent antibody response, and the variability in the antibody response with the antigens used to date. However there have been no serious side-effects noted with the use of hCG. There is the need to find a suitable adjuvant other than tetanus toxoid to bind to hCG. A further problem is the cost of production of the vaccine.

Gonadotropin-releasing hormone (GN-RH), a small peptide, has the capacity of being antigenic when coupled with the appropriate adjuvants [39]. However, GN-RH, which is present in the hypothalamus, has a potential problem. The fact is that GN-RH is the principal hormone controlling pituitary hFSH and hLH release. Attempts to inhibit this hormone could result in a subsequent hypogonadal state that, if indeed it was to be found to be irreversible, would be troublesome.

3.4 Sperm Antigens

There have been a variety of sperm antigens that have been identified for immunocontraception [10, 17, 21, 23]. These are identified by a variety of names. The most prominent antigen at the present time is PH-20 [20, 21, 39]. Other agents have been characterised and named such as fertilin, SP-17, SP-10, and, of course, LDH-C_4 [1]. These sperm antigens have all been investigated in animal species, specifically rodents. Their use as antigens have shown a variable response in terms of their ability to reduce sperm function, motility, or fertilisability. The overall average success rate appears to be on the order of approximately a 70%–80% reduction in terms of their immunocontraceptive activity.

One exception is PH-20, which has been found to have 100% contraceptive effect in a rodent model, and is also reversible [17, 20, 40, 41].

A problem for the human is the possibility that you would need more than one sperm antigen in order to obtain contraceptive efficacy.

3.5 Summary of Current Status

Immunocontraception has been found to be effective, particularly in animal species, where there is evidence of the reduction in the population of wild horses and white tail deer in the western United States using injections of zona pellucida antigens [42–45]. This zona pellucida antigen has also been found to be effective in reducing fertility in elephants [46]. These results hold out a promise for the development of a successful immunocontraceptive for humans.

Although we have practical immunocontraceptive agents that are currently being used in animals as shown above, the development of an effective reversible and tissue-specific antigen for human fertility continues to be elusive. Ongoing work in the immunology of reproduction has raised expectation that an appropriate epitope or antigen can be identified with successful introduction into early preclinical human trials within the next 5–10 years.

Acknowledgements. The author wishes to express his appreciation to Drs. N.J. Alexander, J.C. Herr, and M.J. O'Rand, who took their time to address some of the problems and successes in the field of immunocontraception.

References

1. Feng H, Sandlow JI, Sparks AE, Sandra A (1999) Development of an immunocontraceptive vaccine. Current status. J Reprod Med 44:759–65
2. Barber MR, Fayrer-Hosken RA (2000) Evaluation of somatic and reproductive immunotoxic effects of the porcine zona pellucida vaccination. J Exp Zool 286:641–646

3. Govind CK, Gupta SK (2000) Failure of female baboons (Papio anubis) to conceive following immunization with recombinant non-human primate zona pellucida glycoprotein-B expressed in Escherichia coli. Vaccine 18:2970–2978
4. Tung KS, Ang J, Lou Y (1996) ZP3 peptide vaccine that induces antibody and reversible infertility without autoimmune oophoritis. Am J Reprod Immunol 35:181–183
5. Tung KS, Teuscher C (1995) Mechanisms of autoimmune disease in the testis and ovary. Hum Reprod Update 1:35–50
6. Tung KS, Lou YH, Luo AM, Ang J (1994) Contraceptive vaccine assessment based on a murine ZP3 mini-autoantigen. Reprod Fertil Dev 6:349–355
7. Tesarik J (1995) Targeting the zona pellucida for immunocontraception: a minireview. Hum Reprod 10 [Suppl 2]:132–139
8. Talwar GP (1997) Vaccines for control of fertility and hormone-dependent cancers. Immunol Cell Biol 75:184–189
9. Ramsay AJ, Ramshaw IA (1997) Cytokine enhancement of immune responses important for immunocontraception. Reprod Fertil Dev 9:91–97
10. Alexander NJ, Bialy G (1994) Contraceptive vaccine development. Reprod Fertil Dev 6:273–280
11. O'Rand MG, Lea IA (1997) Designing an effective immunocontraceptive. J Reprod Immunol 36:51–59
12. Prasad SV, Wilkins B, Dunbar BS (1996) Molecular biology approaches to evaluate species variation in immunogenicity and antigenicity of zona pellucida proteins. J Reprod Fertil [Suppl 50]:143–149
13. Stevens VC (1992) Future perspectives for vaccine development. Scand J Immunol [Suppl 11]:137–143
14. Mukhopadhyay A, Bhatia PK, Majumdar SS (1998) Preliminary studies with recombinant chorionic gonadotropin beta- subunit produced in Escherichia coli for use as an antigen in a birth control vaccine. Am J Reprod Immunol 39:172–182
15. Frayne J, Hall L (1999) The potential use of sperm antigens as targets for immunocontraception; past, present and future. J Reprod Immunol 43:1–33
16. Moore HD, Jenkins NM, Wong C (1997) Immunocontraception in rodents: a review of the development of a sperm- based immunocontraceptive vaccine for the grey squirrel (*Sciurus carolinensis*). Reprod Fertil Dev 9:125–129
17. Diekman AB, Herr JC (1997) Sperm antigens and their use in the development of an immunocontraceptive. Am J Reprod Immunol 37:111–117
18. Diekman AB, Norton EJ, Klotz KL, Westbrook VA, Herr JC (1999) Evidence for a unique N-linked glycan associated with human infertility on

sperm CD52: a candidate contraceptive vaccinogen. Immunol Rev 171:203–211

19. Gupta GS (1999) LDH-C4: a unique target of mammalian spermatozoa. Crit Rev Biochem Mol Biol 34:361–385
20. Herr JC, Wright RM, John E, Foster J, Kays T, Flickinger CJ (1990) Identification of human acrosomal antigen SP-10 in primates and pigs. Biol Reprod 42:377–382
21. Herr JC (1996) Update on the Center for Recombinant Gamete Contraceptive Vaccinogens. Am J Reprod Immunol 35:184–189
22. Moudgal NR, Jeyakumar M, Krishnamurthy HN, Sridhar S, Krishnamurthy H, Martin F (1997) Development of male contraceptive vaccine – a perspective. Hum Reprod Update 3:335–346
23. Naz RK (2000) Fertilization-related sperm antigens and their immunocontraceptive potentials. Am J Reprod Immunol 44:41–46
24. Bagavant H, Thillai-Koothan P, Sharma MG, Talwar GP, Gupta SK (1994) Antifertility effects of porcine zona pellucida-3 immunization using permissible adjuvants in female bonnet monkeys (*Macaca radiata*): reversibility, effect on follicular development and hormonal profiles. J Reprod Fertil 102:17–25
25. Lou Y, Ang J, Thai H, McElveen F, Tung KS (1995) A zona pellucida 3 peptide vaccine induces antibodies and reversible infertility without ovarian pathology. J Immunol 155:2715–2720
26. Zona Pellucida Glycoproteins and Immunocontraception (1996) Proceedings of the international symposium. New Delhi, India, 2–5 December 1995. J Reprod Fertil [Suppl 50]:1–198
27. Skinner SM, Prasad SV, Ndolo TM, Dunbar BS (1996) Zona pellucida antigens: targets for contraceptive vaccines. Am J Reprod Immunol 35:163–174
28. Greenhouse S, Castle PE, Dean J (1999) Antibodies to human ZP3 induce reversible contraception in transgenic mice with "humanized" zonae pellucidae. Hum Reprod 14:593–600
29. Talwar GP, Singh O, Pal R, Chatterjee N (1992) Anti-hCG vaccines are in clinical trials. Scand J Immunol [Suppl 11]:123–126
30. Talwar GP (1997) Fertility regulating and immunotherapeutic vaccines reaching human trials stage. Hum Reprod Update 3:301–310
31. Triozzi PL, Stevens VC (1999) Human chorionic gonadotropin as a target for cancer vaccines. Oncol Rep 6:7–17
32. Moudgal NR, Sairam MR, Mahoney J (1985) On the immunogenicity of the beta subunit of ovine luteinizing hormone (oLH beta) and equine chorionic gonadotropin (eCG) in the chimpanzee (Pan troglodytes): effect of antiserum on monkey cycle and early pregnancy. Am J Reprod Immunol Microbiol 8:120–124

33. Moudgal NR (1989) The immunobiology of follicle-stimulating hormone and inhibin: prospects for a contraceptive vaccine. Curr Opin Immunol 2:736–742
34. Moudgal NR, Ravindranath N, Murthy GS, Dighe RR, Aravindan GR, Martin F (1992) Long-term contraceptive efficacy of vaccine of ovine follicle- stimulating hormone in male bonnet monkeys (*Macaca radiata*). J Reprod Fertil 96:91–102
35. Moudgal NR, Murthy GS, Prasanna Kumar KM, et al (1997) Responsiveness of human male volunteers to immunization with ovine follicle stimulating hormone vaccine: results of a pilot study. Hum Reprod 12:457–463
36. Stevens VC (1996) Progress in the development of human chorionic gonadotropin antifertility vaccines. Am J Reprod Immunol 35:148–155
37. Talwar GP, Singh OM, Gupta SK, et al (1997) The HSD-hCG vaccine prevents pregnancy in women: feasibility study of a reversible safe contraceptive vaccine. Am J Reprod Immunol 37:153–160
38. Singh M, Das SK, Suri S, Singh O, Talwar GP (1998) Regain of fertility and normality of progeny born during below protective threshold antibody titers in women immunized with the HSD- hCG vaccine. Am J Reprod Immunol 39:395–398
39. Murdoch WJ (1994) Immunoregulation of mammalian fertility. Life Sci 55:1871–1886
40. Freemerman AJ, Wright RM, Flickinger CJ, Herr JC (1994) Tissue specificity of the acrosomal protein SP-10: a contraceptive vaccine candidate molecule. Biol Reprod 50:615–621
41. Herr JC, Wright RM, Flickinger CJ, Eddy RL, Shows TB (1991) Assignment of the gene for human intra-acrosomal protein SP-10 to the p12—q13 region of chromosome 11. J Androl 12:281–287
42. Kirkpatrick JF, Turner JW, Liu IK, Fayrer-Hosken R (1996) Applications of pig zona pellucida immunocontraception to wildlife fertility control. J Reprod Fertil [Suppl 50]:183–189
43. Kirkpatrick JF, Turner JW, Liu IK, Fayrer-Hosken R, Rutberg AT (1997) Case studies in wildlife immunocontraception: wild and feral equids and white-tailed deer. Reprod Fertil Dev 9:105–110
44. Miller LA, Johns BE, Killian GJ (1999) Long-term effects of PZP immunization on reproduction in white-tailed deer. Vaccine 18:568–574
45. Miller LA, Johns BE, Killian GJ (2000) Immunocontraception of white-tailed deer using native and recombinant zona pellucida vaccines. Anim Reprod Sci 63:187–195
46. Fayrer-Hosken RA, Grobler D, Van Altena JJ, Bertschinger HJ, Kirkpatrick JF (2000) Immunocontraception of African elephants. Nature 407:149

4 Contraceptive Development: Public–Private Sector Alliance

G. Bialy

Contraceptive development research has demonstrated the need for close collaboration between the public and private sectors. The well-documented withdrawal of pharmaceutical industry from contraceptive R&D established the need for the public sector agencies to enter contraceptive R&D. From the beginning there was the realisation that some form of a partnership would have to be established between the two sectors before new products could reach the market place.

Carl Djerassi in his Gregory Pincus Memorial lecture presented at the 1994 Laurentian Hormone Conference stated emphatically that "No new method of birth control will ever reach the general public without the active participation of the pharmaceutical industry. Government or universities are not in the business of bringing new drugs to the ultimate consumer: changing the system would be unbelievably costly and time-consuming." Consequently, during the past three decades most of the new contraceptive products have had their origin in the public sector institutions, while the reaching of the public consumer had its origin in pharmaceutical industry. It is also important to recognise that the so-called pharmaceutical industry component is a heterogeneous lot ranging from one-product companies to multinational giants.

Reflecting on the history of public sector involvement in contraceptive development, we need to remember the development of the first oral contraceptive at the Worcester Foundation for Experimental Biology. For the next decade the pharmaceutical industry became very active in contraceptive research, but unfortunately industrial interests have subsequently subsided. The first public sector agency devoted to contraceptive R&D was the Contraceptive Development Branch (CDB) established within National Institute of Child Health and Human Development (NICHD) in 1969. Its mission was to develop new and improved methods of fertility regulation that could be utilised by men and women primarily in the USA. Following the establishment of the CDB, there followed the establishment of several additional organisations devoted to either in-house contraceptive development or to funding of contraceptive research. Among them in the early 1970s were the

International Committee for Contraceptive Research (ICCR, 1971) of the Population Council, Family Health International (FHI, 1971), Program for Applied Research on Fertility Regulation (PAPFR, 1972), the Human Reproduction Programme (HRP) of WHO (1972), Program for the Introduction and Adaptation of Contraceptive Technology (PIACT, 1976), and the Contraceptive Research and Development Program (CONRAD, 1986). Even before the CDB was established at NIH, the Agency for International Development (AID) provided a sizable grant to the Worcester Foundation for Experimental Biology to explore the utilisation of prostaglandins for fertility regulation.

The public sector has been instrumental in the development of many new contraceptive modalities that industry has translated into commercial products. In the non-federal public sector, examples of these successes include the copper IUD and several versions of Norplant developed by the Population Council, use of antiprogestins for emergency contraception pioneered by HRP, and the contributions made by national research institutions in China and India. In the USA, both the NIH and AID in the federal government have been supporting contraceptive development research and training for over 30 years. These two organisations and more recently a large foundation have provided the bulk of the support for research on spermicides/microbicides. The public sector, with a limited support from the pharmaceutical industry, has also been active in the development of a male contraceptive.

During the early phases of public sector involvement in contraceptive development there was considerable optimism as far as the chances of new product development were concerned. And while the available funding was limited, there was little opposition in terms of the political climate. Unfortunately for the field, public sector funding could not supplant the funds lost as a result of pharmaceutical industry withdrawal from contraceptive R&D. Not only was there a loss of substantial funding, but there was the additional loss of scientific and managerial talent as well as the shrinking of the potential for technology transfer.

It must be recognised from the beginning that the public sector has certain strengths and weaknesses in product development. Its strength stems from the diverse pool of scientific know-how that it can draw on. Thus, many ideas can be pursued without an early preoccupation with marketing of the product. Characteristically, the early pre-clinical stages necessary to establish utility of a product, be it a chemical or device, are conducted with expertise and vigour. In this respect the public sector performance is not much different from that of the private sector. However, as the developmental process progresses through the successive, more complex phases, the importance of participation of the private sector increases. It has been indicated before that fiscal resources and technical and managerial skills critical to guiding a potential product from experimentation to marketing reside primarily in the private sector. At issue is not the need to transfer the technology from one sector to another, but essentially at what point should this transfer take place. There is no simple answer to this question since the technology transfer equation is complex and is driven by divergent forces.

The public sector organisations wish to be involved with the R&D process to a point where the utility of the product can be established. When that specific point is reached will depend on the management of the organisation, availability of resources and the ability to attract a potential commercial sponsor. This would dictate that a dialogue between the two sectors should be on a continuing basis where knowledge of who is doing what and what interests do the respective sectors have, is known. While it is frequently stated that the earliest possible transfer is desirable, this is not necessarily the case for each interaction. One could provide evidence where the public sector could undertake certain steps in the R&D process more readily than the private sector. Thus, for each potential product the situation may vary and the nature of the partnership must be carefully examined. Differences in public-private collaboration will also depend on the precise nature of the public sector institution and the rules and regulations that govern its activities. The public sector is diverse ranging from universities, public research organisations to governmental laboratories and funding agencies. Thus, the nature of the interaction will differ based on policies established at the institutions.

One could provide numerous examples of the two-way collaborations in product development that have existed during the past decade. If anything the trend toward even greater collaboration needs to be established in order to move contraceptive frontiers forward. This will require considerable rethinking concerning the roles that the diverse elements in both sectors must play. It should start with the recognition that there are profound advantages in the interactive process and that both sides have something to gain from the relationship. An element of trust is an absolutely mandatory component. Also, the recognition of the contribution that each side can make must be part of the interaction.

The public sector agencies do not have the resources, nor should they attempt, to play the role of the pharmaceutical industry. The mission of the public sector should focus on the discovery of potential leads that may turn into contraceptive products. The public sector can also play the important role of investigating such areas as vaccine development or male contraception, areas in which the private sector has made only a minimal investment.

The public sector should collaborate with the private sector in the process of strategic planning. Currently, public sector agencies have a tendency to branch out into too many areas of research with the consequence that their resources are spread very thinly leading to inevitable delays. There are numerous examples where development of a lead maybe stretched over a period of two decades. But it is equally important that industry, when it makes the decision to collaborate with a public sector agency, provides a reasonable developmental plan with a time-course that will optimise the delivery of a product to the user. Large multinational pharmaceutical companies are also prone to be slow in their approach to the development of new contraceptive modalities. Even after a product has reached market, there is considerable room for collaboration. There is no doubt that producers of the Norplant device have benefited substantially from the involvement of public sector agencies in post-marketing surveillance and promotion of the specific product. A similar situation exists for the antiprogestin mifepristone.

In calling for the second contraceptive revolution, the Rockefeller Foundation envisioned closer ties between the two sectors. In principle, interactions can be developed that allow for both independence and strong collaboration. We must avoid at all costs any impression that the public sector has become a captive of the private sector. It must also be recognised that while officially interactions involve organisational units, the movement of the machinery depends on people, on leadership that both sectors put forth. Without proper leadership, every initiative is likely to become mired in bureaucratic inertia. The public sector should become more realistic about opportunities that exist and should develop agendas that can be sustained. Carl Djerassi summed up the issue of leadership in the following way: "To implement these priorities into workable solutions, encompassing contraception as well as disease pre-

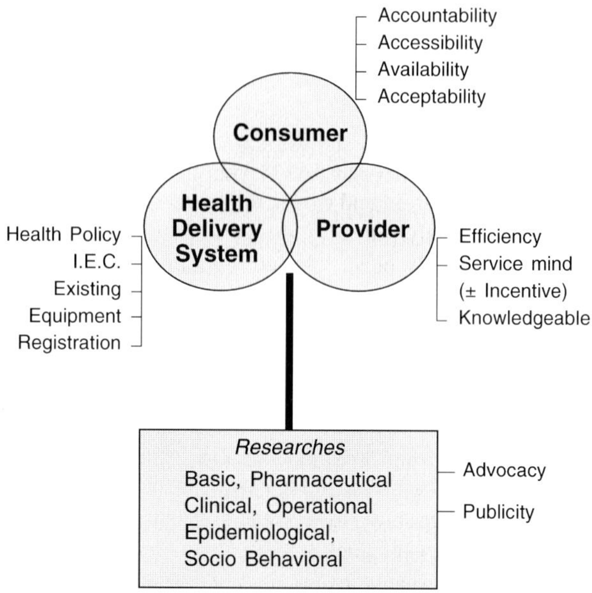

Fig. 1. Marketing and distribution of contraceptives

vention, during the first decade of the next century will require the appearance of another scientist with charismatic and persuasive entrepreneurial qualities similar to those of Gregory Pincus."

In the overall discussion of public–private sector interactions, we need to appreciate the special role of regulatory agencies. The concept of adversarial action should be laid to rest and the spirit of independence with a degree of co-operation be the guiding light. While regulatory agencies have a very specific mission of protecting the public's health, they should be considered as partners in the collaboration in product development.

The time is ripe for implementation of plans that can result in provision of new safe and effective products for management of human fertility (Fig. 1).

5 New Regimens for Female Hormonal Contraception

P.G. Crosignani

In women, contraception can be achieved through hormonal mechanisms that modify critical ovarian or uterine functions, depending on the type and the dose of steroid and on the treatment schedule.

The progestogen-only pill does not consistently reduce FSH secretion so ovulation usually occurs (Landgren and Diczfalusy 1980) and contraception depends on the effect of continuous progestogen on the cervical mucus and endometrium.

The oestrogen component of the low-dose combined oral contraceptives (COC) suppresses FSH secretion while both oestrogen and progestogen inhibit the mid-cycle LH surge (Swerdloff and Odell 1969).

Ovulation is a rare event with COC (1.7%–2.7%) but in the pill-free week interval there is a rise in FSH concentration (van Heusden and Fauser 1999) and if there is any delay in starting the next pill cycle, there is a real risk of ovulation (Killick 1990).

Among the new regimens for female hormonal contraception, COC treatment cycles exceeding 21–23 days and depot preparation are available options.

References

Heusden AM van, Fauser BC (1999) Activity of the pituitary–ovarian axis in the pill-free interval during use of low-dose combined oral contraceptive. Contraception 59:237–243

Killick SR, Bancroft K, Delbaum J, et al (1990) Extending the duration of the pill-free interval during combined oral contraception. Adv Contraception 6:333–340

Landgren BM, Diczfalusy E (1980) Hormonal effects of the 300 μg norethisterone (NET) minipill. Contraception 21:87–113.

Swerdloff RS, Odell WD (1969) Serum luteinizing and follicle stimulating hormone levels during sequential and non-sequential contraceptive treatment of eugonadal women. J Clin Endocrinol 29:157–163

6 Selective Oestrogen Receptor Modulators and Progesterone Receptor Modulators for Contraception

H.B. Croxatto

The potential of selective oestrogen receptor modulators (SERMs) and progesterone receptor modulators (PRMs) as contraceptive agents is worth examining. SERMs are compounds that bind to oestrogen receptors and produce simultaneously agonistic effects in some tissues and antagonistic effects in others. Oestrogen agonistic effects are hard to visualise as playing a role in preventing pregnancy. However, when oestrogens have been used, alone or combined, in very high doses for post-coital or emergency contraception, they have proven to be partially effective. The site and mode of action of the contraceptive effect is unknown in this instance. Tissue-specific antagonistic effects could be enhanced (1) at the level of the cervical mucus, to prevent sperm migration; (2) at the level of the endometrium, to interfere with essential endometrial functions; or (3) at the level of the granulosa cells, to prevent them from acquiring responsiveness to the ovulatory stimulus. While keeping agonistic effects at other levels, these compounds could theoretically become suitable as contraceptive agents.

PRMs encompass progestins, mesoprogestins and antiprogestins. All three classes bind to the progesterone receptor. Progestins have been used for contraception, alone or combined. Mesoprogestins are endowed simultaneously with agonistic and antagonistic properties in the same or different tissues. They should be kept as a separate group, with their own designation, distinct from antiprogestins, since they are not abortifacient. Proper recognition of this fact in their designation is of paramount importance to avoid political obstacles to their development. The pharmacology of mesoprogestins is just beginning to be explored in the human. They have the potential to alter in unforeseeable manners progesterone-dependent processes such as ovulation, implantation and endometrial bleeding. Antiprogestins in turn can completely inhibit progesterone-dependent processes essential for ovulation or for the establishment of pregnancy.

An antiprogestin-progestin sequential regimen that insures ovulation inhibition and good cycle control is currently being tested in a phase 2 clinical trial. When each compound is used for alternating periods of

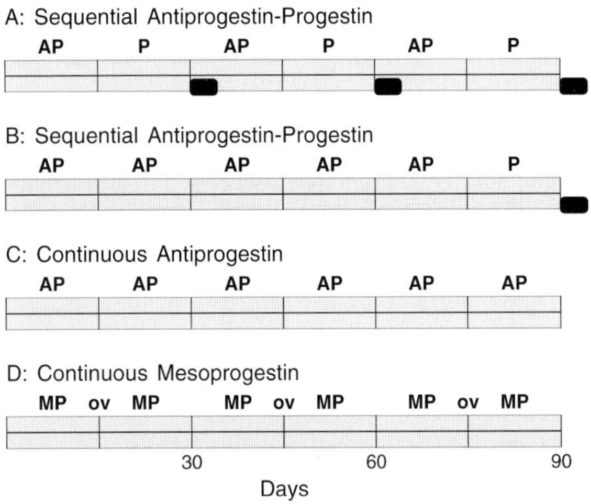

Fig. 2A–D. Four modes of use of PRMs for female contraception. **A**,**B** AP–P sequential regimen that inhibits ovulation. Regular monthly bleeding is achieved in **A** every time the treatment shifts from P to AP. By extending the duration of treatment with AP, as in **B** the frequency of bleeding is reduced to once every 3 months. **C**,**D** Continuous treatment with AP or MP for menstrual suppression has a direct effect on the uterus to reduce blood loss. OV is inhibited in **C** by AP, yet some follicular activity is allowed to provide for systemic effects of oestrogens. OV is maintained in **D** while the MP suppresses the endometrial cycle. *PRMs*, progesterone receptor modulators; *AP*, antiprogestin; *P*, progestin; *MP*, mesoprogestin; *OV*, ovulation

15 days, without interruption, menstrual-like bleeding is ensured at monthly intervals (Fig. 2A). Whereas the extended use of the antiprogestin for a period of 75 days alternating with the progestin for a period of 15 days produces menstrual-like bleeding every 90 days (Fig. 2B). Such decreased frequency of menses, only four times a year, is an attractive option for an increasing proportion of women. Contraception with complete suppression of menses is also attractive for many women. Theoretically, it can be achieved by continuous administration of antiprogestin in an ovulation-suppressing dose (Fig. 2C), or by continuous administration of a mesoprogestin in a dose that allows ovulation to occur (Fig. 2D).

7 Spermicides and Virucides

H.L. Gabelnick

Contraceptive products that protect against the sexual transmission of HIV/AIDS and other STDs, and that can be used by women at their own discretion, are urgently needed. Potential antimicrobial contraceptive compounds should be screened and evaluated for in vitro and in vivo effects of the test agent on:

- Sperm motility
- Other sperm functions
- Fertilisation in rabbits
- Activity against STD pathogens, including HIV

Clinical trials to assess the efficacy of new test agents against heterosexual transmission of STDs and HIV/AIDS continue to face a number of severely challenging constraints, including:

- The need to provide and conscientiously promote the use of condoms and the test formulation, and then to analyse by stratified degree of compliance
- The need to conduct such studies in populations at very high risk of exclusively sexual HIV infection, which is likely to occur only in developing countries
- The very high cost of doing such studies

Finally, as many of the potential agents are not frankly spermicidal but interfere with fertility through other mechanisms, the traditional post-coital screen as the first determination of contraceptive efficacy is not possible. Thus, after initial safety studies, carefully monitored antifertility clinical effectiveness trials are necessary.

8 Menstrual Induction

L. Kovács

Menstrual induction or regulation, a technique originally developed early in the 1970s, is a variant of vacuum aspiration to be carried out up to 6 weeks after the last menstrual period, with a hand-held syringe and a flexible plastic cannula. It was originally seen as ideally suited for widespread use in developing countries because it is simple, cheap and associated with few complications. Additionally, since use of the method does not require a positive pregnancy test, menstrual regulation could possibly be performed without infringing the law in some of the countries where the abortion legislation is restrictive. Attempts have subsequently been made to develop non-invasive, non-surgical methods of menstrual regulation that could be applied in the out-patient department or even by the woman herself. In consequence of their demonstrated ability to stimulate uterine contractions and terminate early pregnancy, the prostaglandins appeared to be a promising pharmacological alternative to mechanical suction. The multicentre trials conducted in the mid-1980s under the auspices of the World Health Organization did indeed confirm that the prostaglandins, and specifically i.m. sulprostone, can be as effective as suction aspiration for menstrual regulation. However, the administration of prostaglandins in therapeutically effective doses was found to be associated with a high frequency of gastrointestinal side-effects and, to a lesser extent, severe abdominal pain, which precluded their routine use. In recent years, the antiprogestational steroid mifepristone has been employed very effectively for the termination of early pregnancy.

Several trials have been carried out with the purpose of evaluating whether a combination regimen of mifepristone followed by prostaglandin can be an effective pharmacological approach to menstrual regulation. The aim of one WHO-conducted multicentre pilot trial was to assess whether a sequential treatment regimen of the antiprogestogen mifepristone (600 mg), followed by the vaginal prostaglandin analogue gemeprost (1 mg), could be used effectively and safely for menstrual regulation. The results of that trial indicated that this drug combination does in fact constitute an effective and potentially useful pharmacological alternative to the currently employed mechanical techniques, with the manual vacuum aspiration procedure foremost among them. Only six failures were registered amongst the 228 women treated, which corresponds to a success rate of 97.4% [1].

There are indications that this regimen can be modified to make it cheaper, easier to administer and more practical and acceptable for widespread use. There is reason to believe that a combination regimen of a reduced mifepristone dose (200 mg) followed by oral misoprostol should be as effective for menses induction, as the treatment approach used in the earlier-mentioned multicentre trial.

The results from that trial further suggested that sequential treatment with mifepristone and a prostaglandin analogue such as misoprostol may be an effective, once-monthly contraceptive for use during the late luteal phase, just prior to the expected menses.

A recent study in Stockholm and Shanghai investigated the efficacy for menstrual regulation of 200 mg mifepristone orally, followed 48 h later by 0.4 mg misoprostol orally [2]. The dose of mifepristone was taken the day before the expected day of menstruation. It was planned that each volunteer would participate for up to 6 months. However, the study was disrupted prematurely due to low efficacy. In 125 treatment cycles the overall pregnancy rate was 17.6% (22 pregnancies) and the rate of continuing pregnancies (failure) was 4.0%. The conclusion was inevitable that late luteal phase treatment with a combination of mifepristone and misoprostol is not adequately effective for menstrual regulation. The combination of 600 mg mifepristone and 1 mg Cervagem for menstrual regulation in women with a menstrual delay of less than 11 days proved highly effective. The reason for the lower efficacy rate for administration before rather than after a missed menstrual period is not known.

Many women would prefer a once-a-month contraceptive method. In a recent survey in Edinburgh, Hong Kong, Shanghai and Cape Town, more than 900 women completed a questionnaire designed to seek their views [3]. At least two-thirds of the women in all four centres were attracted by the idea of a once-a-month pill. In all these centres, however, a pill which worked after implantation (as an early menstrual inducer) was considered unacceptable by over half of the women.

Menses induction by once-a-month pill treatment is not yet practical reality. For the time being, combined injectables seem to be the only effective once-a-month contraceptives.

References

1. World Health Organization Task Force on Post-Ovulatory Methods of Fertility Regulation (1995) Menstrual regulation by mifepristone plus prostaglandin: results from a multicentre trial. Hum Reprod 10:308–314
2. Swahn ML, Bygdeman M, Chen JK, Gemzell-Danielsson K, Song S, Yang QY, Yang PJ, Qian ML, Chang WF (1999) Once-a-month treatment with a combination of mifepristone and the prostaglandin analogue misoprostol. Hum Reprod 14:485–488
3. Glasier AF, Smith KB, Cheng L, Ho PC, van der Spuy Z, Baird DT (1999) An international study on the acceptability of a once-a-month pill. Hum Reprod 14:3018–3022

9 Drospirenone Is Hoped to Diminish Side-Effects of Combined Oral Contraceptives

W. Oelkers

There is a continuing trend to reduce the oestrogen (ethinylestradiol – EE) content of combined oral contraceptives (OC) in order to minimise non-reproductive side-effects of OCs. It is believed, and there is much evidence, that the increased incidence of thromboembolic events in users of OCs is mainly due to the dose of EE, but the effect of EE on the blood coagulation and the fibrinolytic system and on blood vessel walls may be modified by the nature of the progestogen.

Other side-effects may be due to differences between the progestogens contained in OCs and the natural progesterone. Progesterone has an important antimineralocorticoid effect. It antagonises the effect of aldosterone on the mineralocorticoid receptor. In a normal menstrual cycle and during pregnancy, progesterone antagonises the sodium-retaining effect of endogenous oestrogens, which is mediated by stimulation of the renin-angiotensin-aldosterone system. Therefore, extracellular volume and blood pressure are kept relatively normal. The progestogens contained in conventional OCs lack the antimineralocorticoid effect of natural progesterone. For this reason, some predisposed women taking the "pill" may develop arterial hypertension, an increase in body weight and, rarely, oedema. About 15 years ago, Schering developed a new progestogen with antimineralocorticoid properties that we had the opportunity to study intensively in phase 1–3 experiments. Drospirenone is a derivative of 17 alpha spirolactone, which in a daily dosage of 2 or 3 mg inhibits ovulation in healthy young women and leads to a mild sodium loss, and a counterregulatory activation of the renin-aldosterone system. Drospirenone (3 mg) in combination with 30 μg of EE is a new oral contraceptive that, compared with OCs containing levonorgestrel or desogestrel, leads to a slight decrease in body weight and a stable or slightly decreased blood pressure lasting at least 24 months. The new combination will be marketed under the name YASMIN. It is hoped that the development of YASMIN is an important step into the direction of OCs with high acceptability and without significant non-reproductive side-effects.

8 The Elderly and Hormone Replacement

Chair: F. Naftolin
Participants: T. Aso, À. Balogh, K.K. Limpaphayom, B.-M. Landgren, S. Mancuso, H.P.G. Schneider, J.H. Segars, R.S. Swerdloff

1 Introduction

F. Naftolin

Prior to our roundtable there was already ample discussion of the reversal of the demographic trends in recent years. This has very profound implications for the aging population and was referred to at the beginning of our session; Dr. Landgren reminded us of the demographic shifts to aging population.

To set the stage for the discussion to follow, Dr. Naftolin briefly reviewed the lack of a Darwinian evolutionary basis for a specific "Menopausal Syndrome or Response," per se. He described how in the absence of an evolutionary ovarian folliculogenesis there is a recapitulation of the physiological adjustments that occur after loss of ovarian hormones/placental hormones during the reproductive era. These responses may be maladaptive for the post-reproductive woman.

The main issues for the workshop revolved around "What is the potential of the aging population and how can we best serve the aging population of women and men?" Special attention was given to the difference between implications for developed and developing countries. Drs. Aso, Balogh, Mancuso, Limpaphayom and Schneider addressed the needs and effects of various lifestyle changes and the virtues of "hands off vs hand on" ways to prepare worldwide aging populations for the realities of the future, such as better health in the larger, older population than previously envisioned, acute vs chronic hormone treatment, keeping the aging population on the job, the aging population as a resource, etc.

1.1 Moderator's Notes

It is not often that such an august group of principals is drawn together for a single roundtable. Each one of the participants is an expert and able to command their subject without having to deal with the give-and-take of the panel format. It has been said that "moderating a top level panel is like herding cats." In this instance it was especially true in part because of the strictures of time and the fact that our honored guest and maestro, and Madame Maestro, were directly in front of the panel and paying their usual keen attention.

This report has two parts: this partial description of the roundtable's focus and discussions, and the inclusion of prepared remarks that more fully convey specific information by some of the panelists. The latter are presented in an order determined by the moderator to reflect the drift of the discussion. The references accompanying these contributions are far reaching and will serve to further indicate the themes of the roundtable.

"Imitation is the most sincere form of flattery." Oscar Wilde

"Everyone likes flattery; and when you come to royalty you should lay it on with a trowel." G.W.E. Russell, Collections and Recollections, Chap. 23

As a complement to Prof. Diczfalusy's presence permeating these proceedings, the quotations used to punctuate the report were "pinched" from his writings.

"The future is no more uncertain than the present." Walt Whitman

The importance of understanding where we stand today is key. In addition, there are disparate national/regional views of menopause and the remedies employed (vide infra). Dr. Landgren reviewed key issues in the change in the world's demography. In the developed world, the population is aging and there are both opportunities and problems presented. The developing world continues to exceed replacement, with many "hotspots." Dr. Balogh underlined this issue in describing the impact of osteoporosis and the need for new systems of management of health care.

"Poverty is the most widespread, pervasive and intractable disease in the world today." WHO

"The destruction of the poor is their poverty." The Bible, Prov. 10:15

"Man holds in his mortal hands the power to abolish all forms of human poverty and all forms of human life." US President John F. Kennedy

"...that tendency to oversimplification which the human mind displays in all its activities." Arnold Toynbee

The panel largely addressed the developed world and the climacteric. The issue of poverty lurks behind much of what can be accomplished for the developing world's response to aging. Poverty reigns in many parts of the world and makes the response to the elderly rely on custom rather than medicine. As has been so often and eloquently pointed out by our honored maestro, this is not a case of "one size fits all." We must recognize that those absent from the panel include additional individuals from countries where nutrition and public health are not at a level that allows consideration of advanced measures for the recognition and prevention of aging-related diseases. This caveat preceded the considerations of the panel, though it was not the central issue assigned to the roundtable.

"If you can look into the seed of times and say which grain will grow and which will not, speak then to me." William Shakespeare, *Macbeth*, Act I.iii.58

By way of introducing the issues regarding "The Nature of the Climacteric," Dr. Naftolin discussed evidence indicating that there is no (Darwinian) evolutionary adaptation to the lack of ovarian steroids that occurs with aging: Only recently have significant numbers of women lived to the post-reproductive years. Moreover, menopause signals the end of reproduction, sealing off the opportunity for passage to further generations of positive adaptation that could occur by mutation etc.

In the absence of an adaptive response to menopause in the genome, women fall back upon highly successful adaptive reproduction-related responses to the fall of sex steroids that have evolved over the ages. Perhaps this repertoire of adaptive responses is most easily seen during the puerperium, a period when there is a prolonged decrease of sex steroids following a long period of ample sex steroids exposure. During the puerperium, the positive adaptation as a mammalian female is required for successful reproduction and nurturing of the young. However, these "physiologic" responses may be harmful when they are expressed in post-reproductive women. A limited tabulation of these responses, and how they have different effects depending on when they are expressed, is shown in Table 1. The adaptations represented include increased arterial resistance (to maintain blood pressure), mobilization of calcium and lipids for lactation (with attendant bone wasting and lipid elevations in the blood, respectively), loss of reparative sleep (to avoid being surprised by predators and to avoid crushing the suckling infant), radiation of heat to warm the infant (hot flushes) etc.

Dr. Swerdloff elaborated how a similar picture of lack of sex steroids in the aging male is coming to light and indicated that this is an important development since men are also living to the age of gonadal failure. Thus, similar evolutionary implications may be drawn regarding men. Although they may be potent to a late age, their sexual activity and procreation also wane with the fall of secretion of and estrogens with aging.

"All things in life are so multifaceted, contradictory and obscure that we can never be sure about the truth." Erasmus, Praise of Foolishness, Moriae ecomium

Dr. Segars furnished a critique (below) that supports the information about the recognition and treatment of the climacteric.

"We can only see what we have already seen." Fernando Pessoa

Table 1. Responses to falling sex steroids

Adaptive during reproductive era	Affected cell/system	Maladaptive during post-reproductive era
Organ-dependent changes in immune responses	Immunocytes	Failure of immune privilege may ↑ breast cancer and ↓ CNS
Fat up in blood to make milk; maintenance of blood flow to critical organs	Lipoprotein lipase ↑	Atherosclerosis
Sex skin loses elasticity; thinner mucosa	Sex skin function fails	Scarring and genital atrophy
Increased vigilance	Sleep pattern disintegrates	Insomnia; poor performance
Radiation of body heat to suckling infant	Vasomotor control set point changes	Hot flushes
Mobilization of calcium for milk	Cell cycle favors bone loss	Osteoporosis/fracture
Concentration defects; cognitive defects; decreased immune–brain barrier	Central nervous system	Memory defects; dystrophies

Dr. Schneider reviewed the complaints and illnesses that may accompany aging of the climacteric woman. He stressed the need to obtain a careful inventory of symptoms and signs, and offered a standardized assessment that his group has developed and validated for this purpose.

"It is not certain that everything is uncertain." Blaise Pascal

The remaining members of the panel, Drs. Limpaphayom, Aso, and Mancuso then addressed the picture of menopause and treatment from their national perspective. Written contributions from Drs. Limpaphayom and Aso are appended below. The differences between the perception of the climacteric, the remedies, and the national outlook were apparent.

"The scientific revolution is the only method by which most people can gain the primal *things (years of life, freedom from hunger, survival for children)."* C.P. Snow

In summarizing this roundtable, there are several points that come through, especially in respect of the object of our celebration – Diczfalusy and his pursuit of social justice as the salvation of the species:

- To help ourselves we must know ourselves.
- We are in possession of the largest armory of scientific information ever imagined, yet we must have more to survive.
- Education of all is the way to freedom from want and to good health.
- In the context of the climacteric and aging, there is no simple way of describing the universe of the aging population, only the surety that it awaits us and we cannot shirk from our responsibility.

E. Diczfalusy

"Where there is no vision, the people perish." The Bible, Prov. 28:18

Bibliography

Bechmann I, Mor G, Nilsen J, Eliza M, Nitsch R, Naftolin F (1999) FasL (CD95L, Apo1L) is expressed in the normal rat and human brain: Evidence for the existence of an Immunological Brain Barrier (IBB). Glia 27:62–74

Diano S, Horvath TL, Mor G, Register T, Adams M, Harada N, Naftolin F (1999) Aromatase and estrogen receptor immunoreactivity in the coronary arteries of monkeys and humans. Menopause 6:21–28

Gutierrez LS, Eliza M, Niven-Fairchild, T, Naftolin F, Mor G (1999) The fas/fas-ligand system: a mechanism for immune evasion in human breast carcinomas. Breast Cancer Res Treat 54:245–253

Keefe D, Watson R, Naftolin F (1999) Hormone replacement therapy alleviates sleep apnea in menopausal women. Menopause 6:196–200

Mor G, Naftolin F (1998) Estrogen, menopause and the immune system. Journal of the British Menopause Society. Journal of the British Menopause Society 4 [Suppl S1]:4–8

Mor G, Yue W, Santen R, Gutierrez L, Eliza M, Berstein L, Harada N, Wang J, Lysiak J, Diano S, Naftolin F (1999) Macrophages, estrogen and the microenvironment of breast cancer. J Steroid Biochem Mol Biol 67:403–411

Naftolin F, Lavy G, Palumbo A, DeCherney AH (1988) Poissons, grenouilles, femmes et hommes: The appropriation and retention of archetypical systems for reproduction. Gynecol Endocrinol 2:265–273
Naftolin F, Whitten P, Keefe D (1994) An evolutionary perspective on the climateric and menopause. Menopause 4:223–225
Naftolin F (1997) Menopause and Cognition: Short-Term Memory Impairment. Menopause Management 6:17–19
Silva I, Mor G, Naftolin F (2000) Estrogen and the aging brain. Maturitas 38:95–101

2 Hormone Replacement Therapy in Japan

T. Aso

Hormone replacement therapy (HRT) has been widely recognized as one of the efficient methods for the total medical care of the disorders and diseases caused by estrogen deficiency. The indications of currently available HRTs are climacteric symptoms including vasomotor, neurotic and uro-vaginal symptoms, osteopenia and osteoporosis, hypercholesterolemia, and dementia and Alzheimer's disease. The risks and benefits of HRT have been studied extensively.

It has been reported in Western countries that approximately 30%–40% of menopausal women are treated by HRT, but half to one-third of them drop out from the therapy after 6 months of medication. In Japan, HRT was introduced in clinical practice almost 30 years ago, and it has been adapted as one of the medical treatments for climacteric symptoms. The preventive and therapeutic significance of HRT on postmenopausal bone and lipid metabolic disturbances was first recognized about 10 years ago. The percentage of women currently receiving this therapy is about 2% of total menopausal women. These figures are much lower than those of other developed countries. The drop-out pattern is almost the same as that of Western countries. Several reasons have been pointed out why HRT has not been accepted by Japanese women and in clinical practice. First, it has been the general traditional attitude of menopausal problems in Japan to accept the subjective and objective changes in perimenopausal period as the natural events in the aging process of life. Basically, those changes are unavoidable and artificial manipulations should take place. The actual pattern, prevalence, and magnitude of climacteric symptoms of Japanese women are different from those of women in Western countries. It is estimated that the proportion of women who are disturbed in daily activities by severe vasomotor symptoms, like hot flashes, is approximately 25% of total Japanese menopausal women. Since the most common symptom is shoulder stiffness, it seems that the major complaints of Japanese menopausal women do not directly relate to estrogen deficiency. The characteristic pattern of climacteric symptoms of Japanese women is probably modified by the lifestyle including dietary habits, and they have preferred to manage the problems, if any, by improving lifestyle and/or non-HRT management.

As the second reason, Japanese people have been exposed to the rumor that hormones, whatever they are, induce the risk of cancer. In particular, if genital bleeding occurs during medication, most of them easily refuse to continue the therapy. As the general trend, the medical journalism in Japan has not always distributed the information on HRT properly, and they have described the risk of estrogen rather than its benefits. On the other hand, the ordinary people, especially middle-aged Japanese women, do not express their intention of how to be treated. They chiefly depend on the physician when selecting medical care.

As we do not have family doctors or general practitioners (GPs) in Japan, the majority of menopausal women usually consult doctors specialized in internal medicine when they have symptoms and want to have medical care. But only a limited numbers of these doctors are familiar with HRT and are not trained to examine the uterine cytology and breast findings, which are essential for the women given HRT. In addition, a proportion of them believes in the direct causative relation between HRT and endometrial cancer, even though both estrogen and progestogens are included in the therapy, and they tend to emphasize the risks of HRT without any solid evidence.

Thus, it is concluded that the lack of appropriate understanding on HRT by both physicians and patients is the major factor in the limited application and poor compliance of HRT in Japan.

In order to improve the compliance, the awareness of the various problems induced by estrogen deficiency and the role of HRT on menopausal medical care should be promoted to patients as well as to physicians.

Although the physical conditions in perimenopausal period have great influence on the quality of life in the elderly, only a limited number of people are aware of the importance of preventing the increased risk of osteoporosis and ischemic heart diseases resulting from the distinct estrogen deficiency after menopause. But, the preventive health care system covering these diseases has not been fully established in Japan.

At the same time, it is of great importance to establish the consensus that the medical intervention should be selected based not only on the professional standard but also on the patient standard.

References

Aso T, Koyama T, Kaneko H, Seki M (1996) Alternative to hormone replacement therapy for menopausal management: possible role of Kampo medicine. In: Wren BG (ed) Progress in the Management of the Menopause. Parthenon, London, pp 71–77

Aso T (1996) Reproductive health before and after childbearing age: the Japanese scene. Adv Contracept 12:305–308

Aso T (1997) Demography of the menopause and pattern of climacteric symptoms in the East Asian region. Ratnam SS, Campana A (eds) Proceedings of the first consensus meeting on menopause in the East Asian Region. Medical Forum International, pp 24–32

Boulet MJ, Oddens BJ, Lehert P (1994) Climacteric and menopause in seven South-East Asian countries. Maturitas 19:157–176

Lock M (1993) Encounters with aging: mythologies of menopause in Japan and North America. University of California Press, Berkeley

Lock M (1997) Views of Japanese women on menopause: a discussion based on cultural differences with Canada and America. J Jap Menopause Soc 5:53–59

Payer L (1991) International health report. Menopause in various cultures. A portrait of the menopause. Parthenon, London

3 Thoughts on Aging and Osteoporosis

À. Balogh

Health, especially health in old age is one of the greatest assets one can possess. It has even been declared by the World Bank that it does significantly contribute to the wealth of individual nations [1].

Therefore, any wise investment by the society and by the individuals to improve health would result in substantial gains, though they may not be registered at any of the major stock markets.

We are witnessing the changing view of being old because of the rapidly increasing number of elderly and their obvious demand for proper health care. The need for age-adjusted health care exerts a pressure on the providers. How can this problem be alleviated? By changing many paradigms [2]. Being old does not mean anymore inevitably being ill and suffering. Admitting, however, that the chance of suffering is high and increases with age, people might prepare themselves at a younger age to cope with many health problems of aging by finding the right way of living. Our greatest social resource in this search is the contribution by the elderly fellow citizens themselves, whether they are healthy or frail. Because they are experienced and also because they are the most likely to volunteer.

One example of old-age problems is osteoporosis. It is highly relevant to one of the main issues of this Symposium: the complexity of aging and health. Speaking at the end, I am glad to see that nearly all speakers of this session did mention osteoporosis. Based on the outlined trend of world population aging, the incidence and prevalence of osteoporosis and the consequent bone fractures will have a projected exponential growth. In the coming decades, today's health insurance systems may go bankrupt as a result. Primary involutional osteoporosis, with its devastating consequences to the individual, to society, and health care budgets, strikes both women and men, although women are in worse position. When I started studying osteoporosis, more than 10 years ago, this condition was defined by low trauma fracture(s). Today we view it as low bone mass, and an increased chance of fracture, where there is a chance of counteraction. A vast array of cellular, hormonal, and molecular genetic events play an important role in the homeostasis and decay of bones, giving us several chances of timely intervention. This striking change in paradigm took place during the last decade. Another reason why the first fracture must be prevented is gleaned from what large epidemiologic studies have taught us: the first osteoporotic fracture, especially of the spine, is quickly followed by new fractures, like an avalanche. This makes it mandatory to try halt the process of bone decay before the first fracture occurs. Preventive measures can substantially delay its onset and ease the course, thus preventing many of the most feared fractures. Several drugs available now are of major contribution to halt the breakdown of bones. Hormone replacement therapy, theoretically a most natural approach to the osteoporosis treatment, has ample evidence to back it, including the role of gonadal steroids in its etiology and clinical-pharmacological proofs of their efficacy [3]. Other means, perhaps less expensive than drugs, can also significantly contribute to an improved outcome.

Egon Diczfalusy has been warning us of the menace of age-related diseases – one of them is the osteoporosis – as consequences of the worldwide demographic transition [4]. He also draws attention to the need for re-structuring the health care systems and consequently reallocating financial resources to cope with the real public health problems of our current age. I think we are in perfect harmony with him when stating that the solution to health problems of aging can only be managed with the hope of success if elderly people will be active and willing participants of the battle. They represent those primarily affected. Going back to the main issue of this Symposium, my final question: Is there a chance for a healthy aging? The answer may be philosophical or poetic. As I see and feel, Prof. Diczfalusy knows the answer and may share with us the secret at the end of this Symposium in his ever-youthful manner.

References

1. Zagorin A (1994) Real wealth of nations. Time 146(14):146
2. Oldenhave A, Netelenbos C (1994) Pathogenesis of the climacteric complaints: ready for the change? Lancet 343:649–653
3. Balogh À, Bettembuk P (1997) Hormone replacement therapy and prevention of osteoporosis: risk assessment and practical advice. Eur J Obstet Gynecol Reprod Biol 71:189–191
4. Diczfalusy E (1996) The third age, the Third World and the third millennium. Contraception 53:1–7

4 The Challenges of Menopause

K.K. Limpaphayom

4.1 The Asia-Pacific Case

Aging is not a disease, but it can be associated with decreasing physical and intellectual capacities and with increasing disability and discomfort. Some women undergo this transitional period without significant health problems others suffer from progressive deterioration. The diversity in clinical manifestations and health consequences of menopause has evoked various convictions in health perception. The effects of decreased fertility and increased life expectancy also mean that the world's population is growing older. Population estimates for the Asia-Pacific region show that the number of postmenopausal women will increase rapidly in the next 30 years. It is anticipated that, worldwide, twice as many women will reach menopause by 2030 as in 1990 and that the proportion living in developing countries will have increased from 60% to 76%. China alone, where postmenopausal women will make up 17% of the population, will account for 23% of the total. These figures suggest that into the new millennium, the management of menopause in the Asia-Pacific region will pose an even greater health care problem than elsewhere. The perception of menopause in Asian women – it is a commonly held belief that menopause is not a serious life event for most Asian women – has relatively few scientific data to support it. It is common to group Asian women together, but it should be remembered that they constitute a diverse group both racially and culturally. It is, therefore, not unexpected that there has also been some inconsistency in the results of studies on the perception of menopause in different parts of Asia. In Thai society, as well as most other nations around Southeast Asia, menopause is regarded by some conservative groups as a natural change of life not requiring any particular treatment. But on the other hand, physicians consider menopausal endocrine disorders necessary of immediate medical attention and therapy. The environment, lifestyles, language, and culture are crucial in accounting for variations in long-term sequelae of this situation. However, while aging is regarded as being a negative factor in most Western populations, in some parts of

Asia, older people are especially respected for their wisdom and experience.

4.2 The Climacteric Syndrome

There are considerable cultural differences in the reporting of vasomotor symptoms, which may be explained by the meaning ascribed to them and the value of older women in societies, as well as possible dietary, lifestyle, and genetic differences. There has been little variation in the reported prevalence of acute menopausal symptoms in different groups of Caucasian women, considerable cross-cultural variation has been described in both the frequency and in the severity of symptoms. It is a generally held belief that acute symptoms occur less frequently and are less severe in Asian than in Caucasian women, but, although there is considerable evidence to support this view, not all studies have agreed. In a survey of 119 postmenopausal women living in a slum area in Bangkok, 72.3% described vasomotor symptoms, although these were viewed as being a problem in only 29.4% of cases. The differentiation between the presence of symptoms and the extent to which they cause distress is, therefore, clearly important. In another study also conducted in Bangkok amongst women aged 40 years and above, vasomotor symptoms were reported by 80% of those who were rnenopausal, but were also noted by 85.8% of menstruating women. The largest multicenter study in the Asian region also demonstrated considerable differences in the reporting of acute symptoms, but overall, vasomotor symptoms were less common than in Western women. Of particular interest, psychological complaints were more closely related to menopause than were vasomotor symptoms. Overall, most studies suggest that the incidence of acute menopausal symptoms is lower in Asian populations. It has been a commonly held belief that Asian women are more stoical and are, therefore, more tolerant of these symptoms. In addition, it has been suggested that a higher dietary intake of phytoestrogens in Asia may protect women against estrogen deficiency. However, the variation in the reporting of symptoms may also be due in part to methodological differences between the studies. The treatment for the climacteric symptoms in aging groups should be done with a holistic approach. It should be handled by the team of gynecologists, internists, cardiologists, psychiatrists, orthopedic surgeons, rheumatologists, rehabilitation medicine specialists, and clinical nutritionists. Physicians should make more efforts to understand and help women cope with the physical, emotional, and social problems that develop with advancing years. A preventive health program should be made based on the patient's needs and circumstances.

4.3 Osteoporosis

In the Asia-Pacific region, there has been an increase of hip fracture. In reports from Hong Kong in the 1960s, the age-adjusted incidence of hip fracture was between 13% and 30% of that reported in most studies on Caucasians. Since then, however, the incidence of hip fracture has increased in Chinese and in most other populations in this region. This increase has been attributed to greater longevity, reduced exercise, and a change towards a diet that is lower in phytoestrogens. The diet in many Asian populations is also relatively low in calcium, and studies have shown that the dietary calcium intake in postmenopausal Chinese women is less than 500 mg daily. In Thailand, calcium intake for average population is only 360 mg daily. The age-adjusted prevalence of osteopenia and osteoporosis of lumbar spine (L1-L4) are 27.63% and 19.75% and for femoral neck are 37.4% and 13.6% respectively. The cost and lack of availability of many pharmaceutical preparations used in the prevention and treatment of osteoporosis means that the majority of women in the Asia-Pacific region will not be able to choose whether to use one of these treatments. The challenge in osteoporosis prevention will be to determine the minimal doses needed in each age group to pass from global to individual preventive care and to define the strategy for elderly people. There will be an important role for alternatives to classical HRT, such as tibolone, SERM, or bisphosphonates, in the prevention and management of osteoporosis. Optimal non-HRT treatment strategies in osteoporosis prevention depend on age, nutritional status, and physical activity. Women (and men) at all ages should have an adequate intake of calcium and vitamin D. In the elderly, strategies aimed at preventing falls or the impact of falls have to be defined.

4.4 Coronary Heart Disease

Coronary heart disease is an increasing problem in the Asia-Pacific region. Menopause appears to have a similar effect on cardiovascular disease in postmenopausal Asian women as in most other populations. The percentage remains low compared to that in developed countries, considering the size of the population and the rate of increase in the proportion of deaths from circulatory disease. Coronary heart disease may become the most important problem to be faced by postmenopausal women in the Asia-Pacific region. Most women do not know that the most dangerous killer after menopause is not breast cancer, but coronary heart disease: about ten times more women die from a heart attack than from breast cancer. Although cardiovascular mortality is decreasing, morbidity and health care costs are increasing. Interventions to reduce the risk of coronary heart disease by correcting abnormalities of known cardiovascular risk factors in postmenopausal women are warranted both in public health and for the individual.

4.5 Urogenital Aging

Some epidemiological studies have shown an increase of urogenital disturbances in menopause, implicating estrogen deficiency. All these urogenital complaints appear after 2 or 3 years and become stronger with age. Although these disturbances are not life threatening, they affect women's quality of life. Embryological data show that the female genital and urinary systems develop from the primitive urogenital sinus. Different studies have shown that organs of the urogenital trigone have estrogen receptors. There are data that show that decreases in estrogen levels negatively influence the lower urinary tract and genital area. In 1996 in Sydney, at the 8th World Congress of Menopause, Nachtigall reported that postmenopausal women have a variety of troubles in their organs, but that urogenital atrophy occurs in practically 100%. Nobody will die from it, but they will live a miserable life. Problems experienced by these women are urine leakage, an unpleasant odor, urinary infections, perineal rash, and skin infections. Women also have sleep disturbances, restricted social interactions, reduced sexual activity, loss of self-esteem and depression. Employment becomes a problem, and social and private life is changed. Normal genital health for postmenopausal women can be relieved by estrogen therapy. This leads to cessation of genital complaints and, accordingly, to a normal sexual life. In turn, this will improve self-esteem and social and family interactions. Urogenital aging is not life threatening but has a major impact on quality of life in postmenopausal women. Estrogen therapy is the most widely available regimen for alleviation of the negative impact of urogenital aging on quality of life.

4.6 Sexuality After Menopause

Some women may feel their uselessness to society once they become menopausal and may end their active sexual life with the onset of menopause. This misinformation should be corrected. The physical changes that occurred are reduction of production of vaginal fluid, some loss of vaginal elasticity and thinning of vaginal tissues resulting in dyspareunia. The effects of short-term estrogen therapy in improving psychological symptoms, maintaining vaginal lubrication, decreasing vaginal atrophy, and increasing pelvic blood flow in postmenopausal women is well known. However, some patients require more than estrogen alone to improve psychological dysfunction, decreased sexual desire, or other sexual problems associated with menopause. Results from clinical studies show that HRT with estrogens plus androgens provides a greater improvement in psychological and sexual symptoms. Dehydroepiandrosterone, a precursor of estrogens and androgens, could become of practical importance in hormonal substitution in females and males.

4.7 CNS and estrogen deficiency

There is evidence to suggest that HRT positively influences alertness, cognitive function, affective and sexual behaviors, memory, motor activity, pain perception, and well-being in general. HRT has a clinically evident mental tonic effect. It is a more physiological substitute for tranquilizers and antidepressants, which are still used too often to treat the climacteric syndrome. Dementia of the Alzheimer's type has become a major health problem. Some epidemiological studies have shown a reduction in the incidence of Alzheimer's disease in postmenopausal women treated with HRT. Estrogens stimulate the outgrowth of neuronal processes and synaptic connections, with positive effects on neuronal size, number, connectivity, volume, and plasticity. Androgens and progesterone produce many effects in the nervous system. Alterations in the circulating levels of androgens play an important role in the psychological and sexual changes that occur after menopause. However, primary mental disorders are not primarily caused by a deficiency of sex hormones. Therefore, estrogens cannot currently be employed as causative primary therapy for mental disorders in the postmenopausal.

4.8 Conclusion

Most aging women are reasonably healthy and do not need specialized medical care. Emphasis must be on health education and maintenance with particular attention on prevention and early detection of life-threatening conditions. Most of the pathologic changes start years before menopause sets in. The process of health maintenance should start before the actual cessation of menstruation and should be continued until death. Proper counseling about all the changing aspects should include information regarding general health and alteration in lifestyle towards reduction of risks. To reach these goals, the following conditions have to be fulfilled:

- Better education of doctors and paramedics
- A vailability of support groups for menopausal women
- More specific medical counseling
- Improved menopausal center organization to meet women's individual needs
- Access to HRT for women in low socioeconomic conditions

In our aging society, the quality of life of elderly and very old women will largely depend on the ability of society to cope with the economic, social, and medical challenges of menopause.

5 Hormone Replacement in an Aging Population of Women

H.P.G. Schneider

Women tend to see physicians less frequently after 55 years of age. Thus, use of HRT is less common in the age group of 56–65 years. Particular concern in this age group is the need to reduce the risk of chronic diseases such as osteopenia/osteoporosis and cardiovascular disorders. An increasing body of evidence suggests that the beneficial impact of estrogen on the risk of fracture persists only while therapy is continued; long-term treatment is required to reduce long-term risk. Bisphosphonates, which inhibit bone remodeling, have been shown to reduce the risk of osteoporosis and related fractures up to 7 years, although longer-term skeletal effects remain uncertain. Raloxifene is effective in preventing osteoporotic vertebral fractures, but more data are needed regarding hip fractures. Calcitonin, an inhibitor of bone resorption, is effective for preventing bone loss associated with estrogen deficiency and for reducing the risk of osteoporotic spinal fractures. As far as cardiovascular disease is concerned, extensive data from animal investigations and observational studies have shown that HRT has many beneficial effects on coronary heart disease (CHD) risk factors, including favorable alternatives in the lipid profile, vasodilatory effects, and the promotion of angiogenesis. The use of HRT for secondary prevention remains controversial; randomized, controlled trials are under way.

Population aging has become a public health challenge for all the world. To preserve and improve health, women aged 66 years and older should continue to undergo regular screenings and to observe recommendations for healthy lifestyles so as to prevent the development of diseases. Specific, common conditions that must be addressed in this age group include:

- Osteoporosis and associated fractures. Women with osteoporotic fractures require rehabilitation and supportive measures. Pharmacotherapy and lifestyle modifications should be instituted to reduce subsequent fracture risk. Current treatment options for osteoporosis include estrogens, bisphosphonates, calcitonin, and raloxifene. Estrogen replacement therapy and bisphosphonates are regarded as first-line treatments for osteoporosis.

- Secondary prevention of CHD should be aimed at reducing disease progression, preventing future events, and, if possible, inducing regression. Lifestyle modifications and pharmacotherapy can help achieve these goals. Estrogen replacement therapy has been demonstrated to afford protection against cardiovascular disease after cessation of menses. The available body of evidence also supports the use of estrogen replacement therapy (ERT) in women with a previous history or existing cardiovascular disease. Several investigations have shown that HRT does not elevate blood pressure. Therefore, hypertension should be treated as an independent entity, regardless of whether the patient requires HRT. The need for HRT should be weighed separately.
- The acute management of stroke is aimed at minimizing disability and maximizing quality of life. Secondary prevention is targeted mainly towards the control of blood pressure. ERT increases blood flow in the middle cerebral and carotid arteries while also reducing atherosclerosis. Therefore, ERT may be beneficial in women with a history of stroke. Most studies have also shown a decrease in stroke-related complications among ERT users.
- The treatment of Alzheimer's disease (AD) is currently only supportive. New strategies for treating AD remain under study. Experimental evidence has shown that ERT has beneficial effects on cognitive function. Improvement in assessments of memory and cognitive function have been demonstrated, but large-scale multi-center trials are warranted to provide more comprehensive evaluation of this issue.
- The treatment of rheumatoid arthritis is directed towards suppressing the inflammatory process, ameliorating symptoms, and preventing progressing joint damage. The importance of HRT is under investigation.
- The use of HRT may increase the risk of thromboembolism minimally, at a rate of 4 cases per 10,000 women-years, however, in women with previous venous thrombosis, the risk increases to one or 2 cases per 2,000 women-years. When deciding for HRT in a woman with a history of venous thrombosis, it is important to consider the nature of the thromboembolic episode. If the episode occurred during prolonged confinement to bed or for an injury, the patient will probably be at low risk for recurrence while taking HRT.

The health plan for the adult woman must incorporate an individualized assessment of the risk of cancer. Breast cancer, according to several observational studies, has been found increased among HRT users, although this risk never doubles. There is no evidence that HRT may cause breast cancer. Most epidemiological studies fail to be continued for long enough, in order to avoid selection bias as well as bias due to pre-existing disease. Therefore, the question of whether HRT really increases the risk of breast cancer has not been definitively resolved. Breast cancer that develops in women using HRT is more localized and well differentiated and may have a better prognosis than in never-users. HRT is generally not indicated in patients with a disease, although studies have shown no adverse effect of HRT on survival time and disease-free time, but rather reduced mortality. Endometrial cancer develops in women using ERT; progestin opposition is pertinent for equilibrating this risk. In women who have developed endometrial cancer, the use of HRT has not been shown to increase the risk of disease recurrence or mortality. The continuous–combined mode of HRT should be useful. Thus far, no clear correlation has been observed between HRT and the risk of cervical, ovarian, or vulvar cancer. Colorectal cancer has a widely varying incidence throughout the world. This may go from 3.4 cases per 100,000 population in Nigeria, but reaching 35.5 cases in the state of Connecticut in the United States. Approximately 10%–15% of all colorectal cancers are hereditary. Retrospective analyses have shown that the risk of colorectal cancer tends to be low in women taking HRT, although the relationship has been tenuous in some studies. There is no available information on the effect of HRT on the risk of pre-existing colorectal cancer. The incidence is reduced by 50% with exercise. According to International Menopause Society recommendations, age-adapted general health plans are best suited to optimize preventive health care and treatment of age-specific diseases so as to compress morbidity of the aging population.

6 Future Research Directions in Estrogen Action

J.H. Segars

6.1 Introduction

During the twentieth century remarkable advances occurred in science and medicine that will shape the near future. As outlined by Dr. Egon Diczfalusy in recent visionary lectures and publications [1–3], among the most significant developments was the introduction of contraception and the increased longevity enjoyed by human beings. These advances bring into sharp focus the need for effective medical care for aging women, particularly with respect to hormonal replacement therapy to prolong health after natural cessation of ovarian function, or surgical removal of the ovaries. As suggested by Dr. Diczfalusy, satisfactory solutions to the demographic problems facing all providers who care for women throughout the world will be realized only through knowledge generated by clinical and basic research.

The clinical conundrum is to provide replacement therapy to retard aging, maximize health, and yet minimize untoward side effects. For aging women these objectives focus on the steroid hormone estrogen, since estrogens are arguably the most critical products of the pre-menopausal ovary.

Furthermore, estrogens have been proven to have health benefits to aging women after natural cessation of ovarian function. Given the importance of estrogen to aging women, it is useful to summarize the progress that has been made in basic research regarding understanding of estrogen action, and then apply this understanding to the issue of optimal hormone therapy for aging women.

6.2 Recent Advances in Understanding of Estrogen Action

During the last century in general, and the last decade in particular, understanding of estrogen action has advanced through basic research. The century opened with the demonstration that ovaries (estrogen) influenced cancer growth [4] and closed with the understanding that the steroid hormone estrogen acts through at least two modular nuclear hormone receptors which were shown to be present in reproductive tissues (reviewed in [5]). Perhaps not surprisingly, the estrogen receptor was one of the first receptors to be cloned, and this development yielded many insights into the mechanism of hormone action. For instance in the late 1980s and early 1990s the activated estrogen receptor was shown to be a transcription factor that bound to specific DNA sequences. Binding to these estrogen receptor target sites was shown to influence transcription of specific genes [6,7], which in turn led to production of specific messenger RNAs that were capable of altering cell functions, such as growth. Indeed, estrogen and the estrogen receptor often served as a model for the super family of nuclear hormone receptors.

In the past 5 years substantial discoveries have been made in the understanding of estrogen action. A significant advance in thinking followed the report by Gustafsson's group of the estrogen receptor beta in 1996 [8].

An appreciation of the second estrogen receptor clarified some puzzling results of the estrogen receptor "knock-out" (ERKO) mouse [9], and paved the way for BERKO mice [10], as well as mice lacking both estrogen receptor alpha and beta [11]. Cloning and isolation of the estrogen receptors in turn led to the isolation of cofactors that interacted with the receptor to either augment or repress function of the receptor in 1995 and subsequently [12,13]. This advancement was truly remarkable, since this led to the realization that steroid receptors interacted directly with factors that functioned to catalyze histone acetylation [reviewed in 14], and that these intermediary coactivator proteins also were capable of direct binding to RNA transcription factors shown to be essential for RNA production. In keeping with a role for such factors in estrogen action, targeted disruption of such factors, for example SCR-1, has been shown to cause partial resistance to hormone action [15]. Furthermore, structural analysis of the ligand-binding domain of estrogen receptor alpha revealed on a molecular level that binding of an agonist was associated with a conformational change in an alpha helix (helix 12) of the receptor, distinct from the conformation upon binding of a partial agonist [16].

Thus at the close of the twentieth century, estrogen action is understood at a molecular level to a degree almost unimaginable 20 years ago. The improved understanding of estrogen action that has occurred in the past decade has helped promote the development and clinical implementation of pharmacological compounds that were capable of acting as an estrogen agonist in some tissues (such as bone) and an antagonist in other tissues (such as the breast). Specifically, in reference to aging, pharmacologic agents may be targeted to relieve the detrimental health consequences associated with aging and cessation of ovarian function.

6.3 Future Research Directions

As impressive as the advancements regarding understanding of estrogen action are [17], the state of knowledge of estrogen action is far from complete. Research has focused on augmentation of transcription by the estrogen receptor, but not all actions of estrogen in reproductive tissues and the central nervous system involve receptor action as a transcription factor – some occur immediately without sufficient time for transcription of messenger RNA [17,18]. In fact, the estrogen receptor has been shown to be activated by cytoplasmic signaling cascades involving cyclic adenosine monophosphate [19], protein kinases [20], small guanosine triphosphate-binding proteins [21], and growth factors [22], yet an understanding of such pathways is rudimentary at present.

Phosphorylation of the estrogen receptor is surely involved with some rapid response pathways, but it is not yet clear whether all rapid estrogen effects may be explained by phosphorylation. In addition, the specific protein complexes and site of receptor phosphorylation remain unclear. As research into the mechanism of estrogen action has progressed, some very rapid effects of estrogen have been classified as "non-genomic" signifying insufficient time for the response to proceed through RNA transcription [18]. At the close of the century, it is not clear whether it is appropriate to classify all rapid or phosphorylation-dependent estrogen signaling as "non-genomic" in nature.

Rapid actions of estrogen appear to be of clinical relevance, since cardiac, central nervous system, and ovarian estrogen actions appear to involve these signaling pathways. Stated differently, presence of receptor, ligand, and estrogen receptor cofactors is insufficient to explain all physiologic processes. The examples are too numerous to cite inclusively here, but include key central nervous system responses, vascular effects, as well as important in vivo physiologic responses. For instance, in the peri-ovulatory granulosa cells, progesterone receptor is induced in response to the luteinizing hormone surge through an estrogen receptor-dependent mechanism, but in pre-antral and antral granulosa cells both estrogen receptor alpha and beta do not induce progesterone receptor despite high levels of estrogen. Curiously, in this circumstance, the presence of ligand and receptor are insufficient to explain action of the receptor; it is not clear whether a repressor of progesterone receptor gene causes this effect, or whether estrogen action is somehow repressed. A further argument for continued basic studies of estrogen action is that most identified receptor cofactors are expressed widely, and thus the mere presence of the cofactors and proteins acting as coactivators would not appear to explain the differential response of tissues to estrogens, or anti-estrogens. For example, in a study of endometrial cancer-cell lines variably responsive to estrogens, expression levels of coactivators did not vary greatly [23]. Although not demonstrated for the estrogen receptor, progesterone has been reported to directly affect function of the oxytocin receptor, a G-protein-coupled receptor [24]. Collectively, the findings from a number of laboratories around the world suggest that despite advances, our current understanding of estrogen action remains incomplete.

6.4 The Clinical Challenge

At present, the perfect hormonal agent to retard the processes of aging in the menopausal women does not exist. The ideal agent would prevent hot flushes, maintain bone mass, retard development of cardiovascular disease, prove to preserve mood and libido, maintain connective tissue, and would minimize stimulation of endometrial and breast epithelium [25, 26]. A potentially exciting development is the third generation of SERMs, at least one of which appears to act as a pure anti-estrogen [27]. The development of this, and related SERMs, provides evidence that selective modulation of the estrogen receptor is feasible.

For a number of reasons, both medical and socioeconomic, many women throughout the world continue to live without the benefits of hormone replacement therapy after natural cessation of ovarian function, despite the clearly demonstrated medical benefits for the majority of women who may be candidates for this treatment. Menstrual bleeding, to note just one problem, renders hormone therapy unsatisfactory to many women. Other problems, such as concern about promotion of cancer, further reduce the number of aging women that enjoy the benefits of hormonal treatment. While the socioeconomic factors underlying access to medical therapy are addressed, it is precisely the limitations of current medical therapy that argue most strongly for further basic and clinical research on the mechanism of estrogen action.

As the population of women who are candidates for hormone treatment continues to grow, it might be argued that insufficient resources have been devoted to optimization of prevention of the effects of aging in women. This coming challenge has been succinctly presented by Dr. Diczfalusy [1–3]. All scientists and physicians who care for aging women have been greatly aided by the vision of Dr. Diczfalusy. The challenge articulated by him is for basic and clinical research of the scientists of today and tomorrow to focus upon the growing population of aging women, and that active pharmacological research continue in this important and worthwhile cause.

References

1. Diczfalusy E (1997) In search of human dignity: gender equity, reproductive health, and healthy aging. Int J Obstet Gynecol 59:195–206
2. Diczfalusy E (1999) The past, present, and future. Int J Gynaecol Obstet 67:S153–S157
3. Diczfalusy E (2000) The contraceptive revolution. Contraception 61:3–7
4. Beatson G (1896) Lancet 2:104–107
5. Parker MG (1999) Transcriptional activation by oestrogen receptors. Biochem Soc Symp 63:45–50
6. Seiler-Tuyns A, Walker P, Martinez E, Merillat AM, Givel F, Wahli W (1986) Identification of estrogen-responsive DNA sequences by transient transfection in a human breast cancer cell line. Nuc Acids Res 14:8755–8770
7. Evans RM (1988) The steroid and thyroid hormone receptor superfamily. Science 240:889–895
8. Kuiper GGJ, Enmark E, Pelto-Huikko M, Nilsson S, Gustafsson J-A (1996) Cloning of a novel estrogen receptor expressed in rat prostate. Proc Natl Acad Sci USA 93:5925–5930
9. Korach KS (1994) Insights from the study of animals lacking functional estrogen receptor. Science 266:1524–1527

10. Krege JH, Hodgin JB, Couse JF, Enmark E, Warner M, Mahler JF, Sar M, Korach K, Gustafsson J-A, Smithies O (1998) Generation and reproductive phenotypes of mice lacking estrogen receptor b. Proc Natl Acad Sci USA 95:15677–15682
11. Couse JF, Hewitt S, Bunch DO, Sar M, Walker VR, Davis BJ, Korach KS (1999) Postnatal sex reversal of the ovaries in mice lacking estrogen receptor a and b. Science 286:2328–2331
12. Onate SA, Tsai ST, Tsai MJ, O'Malley BW (1995) Sequence and characterization of a coactivator for the steroid hormone receptor superfamily. Science 270:1354–1357
13. Cavailles V, Dauvois S, Lopez G, Hoare S, Kushner PJ, Parker MG (1995) Nuclear factor RIP 140 modulates transcriptional activation by the estrogen receptor. EMBO J 14:3741–3751
14. Edwards DP (1999) Coregulatory proteins in nuclear receptor action. Vit Horm 55:165–219
15. Xu J, Qiu Y, DeMayo FJ, Tsai SY, Tsai M-J, O'Malley BW (1998) Partial hormone resistance in mice with disruption of the steroid receptor coactivator-1 (SRC-1) gene. Science 279:1922–1925
16. Brzozowski AM, Pike W, Dauter Z, Hubbard RE, Bonn T, Engstrom O, Ohman L, Greene GL, Gustafsson J-A, Carlquist M (1997) Molecular basis of agonism and antagonism in the oestrogen receptor. Nature 389:753–757
17. Muramatsu M, Inoue S (2000) Estrogen receptors: how do they control reproductive functions and nonreproductive functions? Biochem Biophys Res Comm 270:1–10
18. Christ M, Haseroth K, Falkenstein E, Wehling M (1999) Nongenomic steroid actions: fact or fantasy? Vit Horm 57:325–373
19. Aronica M, Katzenellenbogen BS (1993) Stimulation of estrogen receptor-mediated transcription and alteration in phosphorylation state of rat uterine ER by estrogen, cAMP, and IGF-1. Mol Endocrinol 7:743–752
20. Cho H, Katzenellenbogen BS (1993) Synergistic activation of estrogen receptor-mediated transcription by estradiol and protein kinase activators. Mol Endocrinol 7:441–452
21. Rubino D, Driggers P, Arbit D, Kemp L, Miller B, Coso O, Pagliai K, Gray K, Gutkind S, Segars J (1998) Characterization of Brx, a novel Dbl family member that modulates estrogen action. Oncogene 16:2513–2526
22. Bunone G, Briand PA, Miksicek RJ, Picard D (1996) Activation of the unliganded estrogen receptor by EGF involves the MAP kinase pathway and direct phosphorylation. EMBO J 15:2174–2183
23. Thenot S, Charpin M, Bonnet S, Cavailles V (1999) Estrogen receptor cofactors expression in breast and endometrial human cancer cells. Mol Cell Endocrinol 156:85–93

24. Grazzini E, Guillion G, Mouillac B, Zingg HH (1998) Inhibition of oxytocin receptor function by direct binding of progesterone. Nature 392:509–512
25. Mitlak BH, Cohen FJ (1997) In search of optimal long-term female hormone replacement: the potential of selective estrogen receptor modulators. Horm Res 48:155–163
26. Leondires MP, Segars J, Walsh BW (1999) The use of antiestrogens in the postmenopausal woman. In: Seifer DB, Kennard EA (eds) Contemporary endocrinology. Menopause: endocrinology and management. Humana, Totowa, pp 179–207
27. Labrie F, Labrie C, Belanger A, Simard J, Gauthier S, Luu-The V, Merand Y, Giguere V, Candas B, Lou S, Martel C, Singh S, Fournier M, Coquet A, Richard V, Charbonneau R, Charpenet G, Tremblay A, Tremblay G, Cusan L, Veilleux R (1999) EM-652 (SCH 57068), a third generation SERM acting as a pure antiestrogen in the mammary gland and endometrium. J Steroid Biochem Mol Biol 69:51–84

9 Concluding Remarks

E. Diczfalusy

Professor Stock, Prof. Raff, Prof. Oettel, dear friends and colleagues, ladies and gentlemen, in the Imperial séance of 7 June 1815, Napoleon remarked that "Men are powerless to secure the future; institutions alone fix the destinies of nations."

Certain institutions may even "fix" the destinies of individuals, albeit those were rarely, if ever, considered by Napoleon. The millennia-old institution of the three wise men may serve as an example. In our modern times, we are constantly facing new realities and in order to meet the new challenges, we are inventing new mechanisms, or – more frequently – reinventing old ones, like the European Union did recently and successfully with the mechanism of the three wise men. To be frank, even I did the same, although more than 50 years ago.

Professor Benagiano mentioned the three wise men who were shaping my scientific career and scientific philosophy; George Ivánovics in Szeged in microbiology, Hans von Euler in Stockholm in classical biochemistry, and Axel Westman, also in Stockholm, in obstetrical and gynecological endocrinology, and I will always remain indebted to them for what they have done for me. However, I learned at an early stage of my career that a good scientist should do things at least in triplicate. Hence, I also had another triumvirate of wise men at the University of Edinburgh. I have learned steroid chemistry from Guy Marrian, statistics from Jack Gaddum and bioassay statistics from David Finney. They had no official relationship to me; it was only spontaneous generosity and friendship that persuaded them to invest an enormous amount of their time into my extremely informal training.

Against this background, it is easy to see that I have a very special place in my heart for Edinburgh and its University. If you would be interested in further details, please consult the chairman of our second Round Table Discussion.

Last, but not least, I also managed to have a third triumvirate of wise men here in Berlin, Profs. Stock, Raff and Oettel. What have they done for me? You have seen it today. They have organized an incredible Symposium with outstanding scientists whom I respect very much indeed. They have brought here from the different corners of the world many of my former students, now old professors, and I must tell you that it was a very special and unique pleasure to listen to these grown-up youngsters. However, the three wise men of Berlin have done even more for us; they have enabled us to have a family reunion here. It is certainly no minor feat, since the last time we had the whole family together was in Rönninge, 30 years ago on the occasion of my 50th birthday. For all this, my very special thanks go to the three wise men of Berlin.

I think it was Aldous Huxley who said that most human beings have an almost infinite capacity for taking things for granted, and I certainly belong to this category. During half a century I took it for granted that it was the natural order of things that my wife should write all my manuscripts, that she should correct my atrocious English, that she should help me with editing, in short that she should do everything for me. In fact, I could never have managed it without her help. Strangely enough, I just couldn't find a suitable public occasion during 50 years to thank her for all this. Thanks to the three wise men of Berlin, I have that occasion here and now, and I would like to express my sincere thanks for providing me with this opportunity.

The question is then, how should I thank you for all this? In 1950, when I first went to London, which was incredibly exciting for someone who spent the war years in Hungary, I realized that English is a most sophisticated language, so I started learning it from the most authentic sources, the "cabbies", the cab drivers. It worked like this: in case you would undertip the cabbie, he would say "Thanks!" It sounded almost like a stroke with a whip. If the tipping was a little bit better, but still not entirely to his satisfaction, the driver would say "Thank you!" In case you were more generous and your tipping adequate, he would say "Thank you very much!" Finally, if he received something highly above the expectations of his most rosy dreams, something he had never hoped for, he would then say "Thank you very much, sir!"

So, Prof. Stock, Prof. Raff, Prof. Oettel, thank you very much, sirs!

Some 350 years ago, the famous Swedish Statesman, Axel Oxenstierna remarked that "at 50 you begin to be tired of the world, and at 60 the world is tired of you." The logical question is then, but what about 80? And now, ladies and gentlemen, we are touching some very sensitive nerves.

Several approaches are open to exploration, like that used by Chandler Harris some 100 years ago, who said – almost in a bragging way – "I am in the prime of senility." Another approach is that you refuse to retire and remain professionally active, in which case you are expected to follow your historical role and preach pessimism. If – at the age of 80 – you don't preach pessimism, something is wrong with you.

Well, I don't preach pessimism, I never was a pessimist. Rather, I followed the principles of Clarence Darrow. Who was Clarence Darrow? Few people would know him today. He was a famous lawyer in Boston in the 1930s. When he celebrated his 70th birthday, he remarked: "At 20, a man is full of fight and energy; he wants to reform the world. At 70, he still wants to reform the world, but he knows that he can't." And at 80, I still want to reform the world and I also know that I can't. However, I also know that your students and the students of those students can and will, because I profoundly believe that it is possible to improve the human condition and that the best way of doing it is through research. I am also convinced that doing research provides you with a very meaningful life.

Strangely enough, at 80 you are also expected to be wise. I really don't know why; maybe it is one of those widely believed misconceptions... indeed, there are so many of them. Thus, your colleagues claim that they are interested in knowing what you have learned during a long lifespan; what are the pillars of your wisdom to be transmitted to the next generation.

In the 1920s, I think it was in 1926, Lawrence of Arabia published his impressive book: *The Seven Pillars of Wisdom.* Even I was impressed...by the title. I never read the book. However, I felt that seven pillars are just too much for me and, in order not to overdo it, it is better to try it only with three. Even that is a big order.

What are then the three pillars; the advice I would like to convey to the next generation?

The first comes from T.S. Eliot's Choruses from *The Rock* (1934): "Where is the Life we have lost in living?/Where is the wisdom we have lost in knowledge?/Where is the knowledge we have lost in information?"

In fact, in these days of "information revolution" it may be useful to remind ourselves that information is no knowledge, unless it is critically assessed and systematized in order to let it form a part of the body of existing knowledge. And knowledge is no wisdom, unless it is used to improve the human condition. To develop a revolutionizing new hydrogen bomb and other modern means of destruction constitutes no wisdom; to develop a new drug to alleviate suffering and to improve the quality of life of generations to come is real wisdom.

It follows from this definition that by far the best way to attain wisdom is to conduct research. Hence research is my first pillar of wisdom.

Also, the second advice is based on a poem of T.S. Eliot: "The East Coker" in *Four Quartets* (1940): "The only wisdom we can hope to acquire/Is the wisdom of humility: humility is endless."

And in this context I feel it worth to remember a statement from Jules Renard's *Journal* (1909) that there is false modesty, but there is no false pride.... Thus, humility is my second pillar of wisdom.

And the third one? I call it the "infinite wisdom of hope" because I am convinced that – in addition to humility – there is also another wisdom we can hope to acquire and that is hope itself. I am also convinced that all of us are the prisoners of hope and that hope is the quintessence of the human condition. That is why hope is my third pillar of wisdom.

Ludwig Wittgenstein's *Tractatus Logico-philosophicus* carries a single motto in which Kürnberger says that "whatever a man knows, whatever is not mere rumbling and roaring that he has heard, can be said in three words." Maybe the three pillars above might qualify for those three words: *research*, *humility* and *hope*.

Subject Index

Ernst Schering Research Foundation Workshop

Editors: Günter Stock
Monika Lessl

Vol. 1 *(1991)*: Bioscience⇋Society – Workshop Report
Editors: D. J. Roy, B. E. Wynne, R. W. Old

Vol. 2 (1991): Round Table Discussion on Bioscience⇋Society
Editor: J. J. Cherfas

Vol. 3 (1991): Excitatory Amino Acids and Second Messenger Systems
Editors: V. I. Teichberg, L. Turski

Vol. 4 (1992): Spermatogenesis – Fertilization – Contraception
Editors: E. Nieschlag, U.-F. Habenicht

Vol. 5 (1992): Sex Steroids and the Cardiovascular System
Editors: P. Ramwell, G. Rubanyi, E. Schillinger

Vol. 6 (1993): Transgenic Animals as Model Systems for Human Diseases
Editors: E. F. Wagner, F. Theuring

Vol. 7 (1993): Basic Mechanisms Controlling Term and Preterm Birth
Editors: K. Chwalisz, R. E. Garfield

Vol. 8 (1994): Health Care 2010
Editors: C. Bezold, K. Knabner

Vol. 9 (1994): Sex Steroids and Bone
Editors: R. Ziegler, J. Pfeilschifter, M. Bräutigam

Vol. 10 (1994): Nongenotoxic Carcinogenesis
Editors: A. Cockburn, L. Smith

Vol. 11 (1994): Cell Culture in Pharmaceutical Research
Editors: N. E. Fusenig, H. Graf

Vol. 12 (1994): Interactions Between Adjuvants, Agrochemical and Target Organisms
Editors: P. J. Holloway, R. T. Rees, D. Stock

Vol. 13 (1994): Assessment of the Use of Single Cytochrome P450 Enzymes in Drug Research
Editors: M. R. Waterman, M. Hildebrand

Vol. 14 (1995): Apoptosis in Hormone-Dependent Cancers
Editors: M. Tenniswood, H. Michna

Vol. 15 (1995): Computer Aided Drug Design in Industrial Research
Editors: E. C. Herrmann, R. Franke

Vol. 16 (1995): Organ-Selective Actions of Steroid Hormones
Editors: D. T. Baird, G. Schütz, R. Krattenmacher

Vol. 17 (1996): Alzheimer's Disease
Editors: J.D. Turner, K. Beyreuther, F. Theuring

Vol. 18 (1997): The Endometrium as a Target for Contraception
Editors: H.M. Beier, M.J.K. Harper, K. Chwalisz

Vol. 19 (1997): EGF Receptor in Tumor Growth and Progression
Editors: R. B. Lichtner, R. N. Harkins

Vol. 20 (1997): Cellular Therapy
Editors: H. Wekerle, H. Graf, J.D. Turner

Vol. 21 (1997): Nitric Oxide, Cytochromes P 450,
and Sexual Steroid Hormones
Editors: J.R. Lancaster, J.F. Parkinson

Vol. 22 (1997): Impact of Molecular Biology
and New Technical Developments in Diagnostic Imaging
Editors: W. Semmler, M. Schwaiger

Vol. 23 (1998): Excitatory Amino Acids
Editors: P.H. Seeburg, I. Bresink, L. Turski

Vol. 24 (1998): Molecular Basis of Sex Hormone Receptor Function
Editors: H. Gronemeyer, U. Fuhrmann, K. Parczyk

Vol. 25 (1998): Novel Approaches to Treatment of Osteoporosis
Editors: R.G.G. Russell, T.M. Skerry, U. Kollenkirchen

Vol. 26 (1998): Recent Trends in Molecular Recognition
Editors: F. Diederich, H. Künzer

Vol. 27 (1998): Gene Therapy
Editors: R.E. Sobol, K.J. Scanlon, E. Nestaas, T. Strohmeyer

Vol. 28 (1999): Therapeutic Angiogenesis
Editors: J.A. Dormandy, W.P. Dole, G.M. Rubanyi

Vol. 29 (2000): Of Fish, Fly, Worm and Man
Editors: C. Nüsslein-Volhard, J. Krätzschmar

Vol. 30 (2000): Therapeutic Vaccination Therapy
Editors: P. Walden, W. Sterry, H. Hennekes

Vol. 31 (2000): Advances in Eicosanoid Research
Editors: C.N. Serhan, H.D. Perez

Vol. 32 (2000): The Role of Natural Products in Drug Discovery
Editors: J. Mulzer, R. Bohlmann

Vol. 33 (2001): Stem Cells from Cord Blood, In Utero Stem Cell Development, and Transplantation-Inclusive Gene Therapy
Editors: W. Holzgreve, M. Lessl

Vol. 34 (2001): Data Mining in Structural Biology
Editors: I. Schlichting, U. Egner

Vol. 35 (2001): Stem Cell Transplantation and Tissue Engineering
Editors: A. Haverich, H. Graf

Supplement 1 (1994): Molecular and Cellular Endocrinology of the Testis
Editors: G. Verhoeven, U.-F. Habenicht

Supplement 2 (1997): Signal Transduction in Testicular Cells
Editors: V. Hansson, F. O. Levy, K. Taskén

Supplement 3 (1998): Testicular Function:
From Gene Expression to Genetic Manipulation
Editors: M. Stefanini, C. Boitani, M. Galdieri, R. Geremia, F. Palombi

Supplement 4 (2000): Hormone Replacement Therapy and Osteoporosis
Editors: J. Kato, H. Minaguchi, Y. Nishino

Supplement 5 (1999): Interferon:
The Dawn of Recombinant Protein Drugs
Editors: J. Lindenmann, W.D. Schleuning

Supplement 6 (2000): Testis, Epididymis and Technologies in the Year 2000
Editors: B. Jégou, C. Pineau, J. Saez

Supplement 7 (2001): New Concepts in Pathology and Treatment of Autoimmune Disorders
Editors: P. Pozzilli, C. Pozzilli, J.-F. Kapp

Supplement 8 (2001): New Pharmacological Approaches to Reproductive Health and Healthy Ageing
Editors: W.-K. Raff, M. F. Fathalla, F. Saad

This series will be available on request from
Ernst Schering Research Foundation, 13342 Berlin, Germany